A
PHILOSOPHY
OF
DIRT

A PHILOSOPHY OF DIRT

Olli Lagerspetz

REAKTION BOOKS

Dedicated to the memory of my parents, with love and gratitude

Published by
Reaktion Books Ltd
Unit 32, Waterside
44–48 Wharf Road
London N1 7UX, UK
www.reaktionbooks.co.uk

First published 2018

Copyright © Olli Lagerspetz 2018

Printed and bound in Great Britain by
TJ International, Padstow, Cornwall

A catalogue record for this book is available from the British Library

ISBN 978 1 78023 918 7

Contents

PREFACE

Wed
5/29/19

The beginnings of this work on dirt go back to my time in Wales
where in 1992, at a young age, I had been appointed lecturer of
philosophy at the University of Wales, Swansea. I quickly realized,
however, that a book of this kind must be written in the author's
first language – in my case, Swedish or Finnish – not Philosophical
English. To start with, 'dirt' is not equivalent to the Swedish *smuts*
– which would be the usual dictionary translation – and in this
general domain quite a few other words, too, would fare badly in
a literal translation. Our concepts of dirt, hygiene and living on
the whole exhibit considerable variation locally, regionally and in
terms of social class, even after years of commerce and migration
within the cultural space of the global West.

When the question of producing a translation of my Swedish
book was brought up, the very reasons that made me originally use
Swedish and not English prompted me to take on the work myself.
Instead of translating, I saw the need to rewrite. My first analysis of
the conceptual web of dirt and cleanliness had taken its starting
point in the self-evident linguistic and social milieu of my upbring-
ing. In order to render the same ideas in a new language, emphases
had to be placed differently and sometimes the whole main line of
argument had to be drawn in a different way. This also meant that
new literature had to be consulted and new debates considered.
Moreover, after the publication of my Swedish book there has been
a steady and increasing flow of relevant new research.

The importance of cultural differences even within (relatively)
united Europe dawned on me at the latest in December 1995, when

Dirt — Cleanliness Binary

our first child saw the light of day in the newly erected Singleton Hospital in Swansea. Singleton was a beautiful, well organized place with high hygienic standards, friendly staff and ingenious details to make life easier for women on the eve of childbirth – a real tribute to the National Health Service after years of Thatcherism. But one detail seemed to confirm in my mind the European stereotype of Britons as inveterate Victorians, inordinately fond of bathtubs, lukewarm water and cosy interiors but otherwise with a doubtful sense of hygiene. We were shown into the delivery room, where the floor was adorned with a carpet. A carpet. I am willing to trust the hospital staff to keep everything perfectly clean, but carpets in delivery rooms are not to be thought of in the Nordic countries.

If I were to sum up the ideas in this book in a few bullet points, a central one would be that the question 'What is dirt?' is closely connected to the question 'What is a thing, what is an ordinary object?' And *that* question can be answered only by describing what it means to *live* with things. Human beings and things have developed together and therefore one can only make sense of any of them by thinking of them together. Like a raspberry worm that lives *in* and *from* its berry home and its berry world, the human being lives in a world of things. The German thinker Oswald Spengler remarks in 1931 that 'the earliest traces of man and his tools are the same age'. It is impossible to imagine the fully developed human hand as active even for a short while without the existence of tools. 'Just as the tool was shaped in conformity with the hand, conversely *the hand arose from the shape of the tool*.'[1] My suggestion is that this symbiosis of man and thing also gives us the concept of dirt as we know it.

The existing theoretical debate on dirt has, however, focused on another question: of whether soiling is a real quality of the environment or merely – as most authors would have it – a subjective idea projected on reality by human consciousness.[2] I argue that the question, which falls within the overarching philosophical 'realism vs antirealism' debate, is meaningless in this general form. In order to address questions about the nature of human access to reality we need to be told of the specific worries and situations that prompt the questions.

I would love to conclude by saying that this work is, of course, just a beginning and that others will no doubt take up my ideas and carry them further. But for one thing I believe I have made more than just a beginning. More importantly, I believe it is pointless in philosophy to look for work for others to do. Where philosophy is going next we simply do not know. It goes wherever *we* take it; you and I and every thinking person – together.

Opposing Ideas/Concepts Are Used To Frame/Classify/Define Issues From Different Ends of Political/Intellectual/Racial/Social/Cultural/Financial Spectrum. Social Issues Are Framed by Public Intellectual, Media Types And Presented To The Public In A Way that Citizens Can Engage The Issue By Placing Themselves Somewhere Along The Continuum Sliding (At The Extremes Or In The Middle). Societal Leaders (Lawyer Politicians, Celebrities, Media Types) Also Position Themselves Somewhere On The Continuum That Will Enhance Their Reputations + Give Them Votes, Money + Power. Am. Society Is Composed of Many Diverse Individuals + Groups of People Who Engage, React, Accept, Reject, Tolerate, In Mostly Egocentric, Different Issues Self-Serving Ways. Due To Multiple Competing Interests, It Is Impossible To Bring Am. Society Together For The Common Greater Good.

PART I

THE PHILOSOPHICAL LANDSCAPE OF 'DIRTY' AND 'CLEAN'

A 'thing in itself', just as perverse as a 'sense in itself', a 'meaning in itself'. No 'facts in themselves' exist, for one must always give them sense before they can be 'facts'.

The question 'What is it?' is a determination of sense as seen from the point of view of something else. The 'essence', 'real nature', is something perspectival and it already presupposes a plurality. At the bottom there is always 'What is it for me?' (for us, for everything living, etc.) . . . In brief: The essence of a thing is one more opinion about the 'thing'. Or rather: 'it counts as', is the real 'it is', the one and only 'it is'.

Nietzsche, *The Will to Power*[1]

ONE

Dirt in Philosophy and Culture

A main source of our failure to understand is that we
do not *command a clear view* of the use of our words.
– Our grammar is lacking in this sort of perspicuity. A
perspicuous representation produces just that understanding which consists in 'seeing connexions'. Hence
the importance of finding and inventing *intermediate
cases*. The concept of a perspicuous representation is of
fundamental significance for us. It earmarks the form of
the account we give, the way we look at things. (Is this
a 'Weltanschauung'?)

Wittgenstein, *Philosophical Investigations*[1]

Homo sordidus: the dirty and clean animal

Homo sapiens is also *Homo sordidus* – not merely the rational
animal but also the dirty (and clean) animal, the animal whose life
is in many ways regulated by ideas of the dirty and the clean.[2] Judging from our current state of knowledge, clean and dirty – like holy
and profane, familiar and unfamiliar, Yes and No – constitute an
organizing principle that is universally applicable and possible to
find in every human society in some form at least. In its ubiquity,
it is similar to Giambattista Vico's universal triad of religion,
marriage and funeral, or of T. S. Eliot's 'birth, copulation and death'.[3]
    The existing anthropological material looks compelling enough.
Nevertheless I believe the important thing is not the apparent fact
that certain customs prevail universally, but rather our expectation

of *finding* that universality. It does not appear impossible, for instance, that there might be a culture somewhere in which the concept of *soup* is unknown; but we could not even imagine finding one where no trace is to be seen of concepts like right and wrong, true and false, family, religion, funeral – or of dirty and clean. And please note that this is not because human nature somehow unfailingly excludes such a possibility, but simply because the existence of a human community does not *appear possible* for us outside certain limiting notions. 'If they have no idea of *that* – then what *can* they have an idea of?' Thus while we expect to find different degrees of tolerance of dirt and various cleaning methods in use in different cultures, we could only shake our heads at the idea of discovering a culture where the categories of clean and dirty are completely missing. We would either doubt the factual account or we would object that it is surely not anything we would call a culture, but something else: a temporary group of shipwrecked, confused individuals.[4]

The question concerning the essence of human culture divides into three further issues: what does actually happen in human societies?; what can imaginably happen?; finally: where are the limits of what we would be prepared to call 'human culture'? In writing this book I have above all had the third issue in mind. It is not as if certain universals always stay put, a riverbed in the shifting stream of human cultural expressions.[5] Instead, our *questioning* about human ways of life guides our understanding in ways that make the universals appear. But we – you and I – are also human. Looking at how humans look at other humans will also tell us a great deal about what manner of beast the human being is.

This can obviously also be applied to how we look at the categories of clean and dirty. Suppose we meet someone who appears to be devoid even of a rudimentary sense of cleanliness. We would not only see her state as deeply disquieting, but would think that an essentially human quality is missing in her – more so than in the case of deficiencies in the area of purely intellectual faculties. Let us here simply remember the role of these considerations in the shaping and un-shaping of human communities. George Orwell famously remarked that it is possible to develop friendship with someone who disagrees with you, but not with someone with a bad smell. And if you ever want to agitate for genocide, you are well advised to start by depicting the target group as dirty and hence as already standing in part outside humanity.

Facts as such can neither confirm nor disconfirm the existence of an unchangeable human nature, because they do not exclude changes in the future or in a past yet undisclosed. What is possible, however, is to look at our *expectations* concerning human nature. Human culture seems completely unthinkable without the categories of the dirty and the clean. On the other hand, our very familiarity with these categories may be a reason why they might be difficult to get to focus. As Ludwig Wittgenstein has remarked, 'the aspects of things that are most important for us are hidden because of their simplicity and familiarity'.[6] We have no record of who was the first to discover water, but we may be reasonably sure it was not the fish.

On the philosophy of something, and, in particular, of dirt

Why add one more work to the already existing library of treatments of dirt and impurity? Is there some good philosophical reason beyond the obvious freak appeal?

The distinction between clean and dirty occurs in every culture but, as far as I am aware, so does the use of fire. Yet we do not seem to be in need of a specific 'philosophy of fire' any more than of 'a philosophy of teacups and of bald-headed stationmasters' – to quote R. G. Collingwood's notes on 'the idea of a philosophy of something'.[7] Collingwood's claim was that philosophy (as opposed to, for instance, ethnology) deals only with concepts that are in principle applicable to *everything* that exists or everything we think and do. Hence there is no philosophy of teacups whereas, for instance, the concepts of thought, action, art, science and history are proper subjects for philosophy. The universality of fire use in human culture, however, seems *accidental* in a way that concepts of clean and dirty are not. Human beings might be able to cater to their needs of heating, cooking and protection by some other means. In contrast – as I will argue later on in more detail – the concepts of clean (pure) and dirty (polluted) carry the potential of being applied everywhere as soon as there is culture; as soon as there is systematic transformation of nature into man-made reality. Dirty and clean are 'transcendentals' in Collingwood's sense; we do not extract these concepts from some specific class of things but they are rather something that we may apply to all reality.[8] Thus the philosophical study of the conceptions of dirt would be philosophy – philosophy of culture, philosophical anthropology – *from the point of view* of dirt.

This kind of study is particularly instructive for one specific reason. Philosophy works with conventionally established dichotomies, such as the mental *versus* the material, factual vs normative, objective vs subjective. The concept of dirt seems to be one that falls between every philosophical stool imaginable. For instance, descriptions of dirt and how it attaches to objects are quite obviously descriptions of material reality. And yet 'dirt' is not a concept of *physics* even though physics is supposed to be *the* science of material reality. Let me simply suggest at this point that we stop trying to force round blocks into square openings.

The central problem is that our present intellectual culture encourages a simplistic understanding of 'matter'. It may be difficult to keep in mind that our manifold conceptions of 'the material' are not identical with the concepts of physics but that they, too, are *sui generis*. It is legitimate to approach material things, not only from the point of view of the physical sciences, but from what one might call the perspective of human existence.

What, then, about the retort that, regardless of any subjective perspective on things, *reality* is one and only, and the question of what really exists is simply a scientific question?

These kinds of dictum have a surface appeal but it is perhaps not quite obvious what they mean. That natural science on the whole has got things right is easily assented to, at least if we add that the state of the art in science is constantly changing, that different natural sciences are not all the same and that other sciences (the human and social sciences) are legitimate investigations about phenomena that fall outside the framework of natural science. In addition, non-scientific activities such as art, literature and religion may also give us valuable insights about reality. The sentence that there is 'one' reality is not so much wrong as impenetrable. 'Realities' are not *things* like apples, and unlike the giant panda, you cannot try to keep track of how many there are, perhaps one day to be horrified to learn that only one is left. 'Reality is one' is a slogan, a call to a fight, and beneath the impenetrable surface a much more accessible claim is offered: that philosophy as we know it is *dead*, and so is religion, literature and every other kind of intellectual pursuit except the most dulling routines of empirical science. And that may well be the case, at least in the lives of the persons who put forward the slogan.

The marginal status of dirt in philosophy and science today does not seem to be due to mere prudery. It reflects a certain approach to ontology, or the nature of reality, commonly embraced in modern theoretical thought. But as we will see, questions about the nature of dirt were influential in the original shaping of the ontology of Western philosophy and science. Thus the current re-emergence of dirt as a philosophical topic is not a radically new development but marks a healthy return to a less one-sided philosophical diet.[9]

The dirt boom and art wars: Andres Serrano
and *Piss Christ*

Dirt is 'in' – as anyone working in the culture sector must know by now. Every gallery with a minimum of self-respect exhibits at least a few objects of 'abject' materials – scraps of meals, sperm, menstrual blood and so on – even though the market is not quite ripe for, say, replicas of Damien Hirst's bisected dead cow to be widely used by home decorators. Seen merely as a picture, Andres Serrano's *Piss Christ* would certainly be better suited to hang over Granny's front room sofa. The photo (from 1987), with sunrays lighting on a lonely crucifix floating in brownish yellow, has a distinct feel of Rembrandt – as long as we overlook the fact that the wonderful haze is due to the urine in which the crucifix is submerged.

Controversies about *Piss Christ* may have started from the fear of hurting the feelings of *the general public*. Should an angry member of the general public show up in real life, the artist and the artwork will have established their reputation as *controversial*. And, since the general public by definition must count as aesthetically retarded, the controversial status of the artwork, once confirmed, becomes a guarantee of its relevance – aesthetically, philosophically or politically. In the best case this is enough to secure wider publicity. Readers of news will have the pleasure of learning in numerous instalments how it is sabotaged, accepted or denied entry in various galleries and countries. This is an artistic war of attrition where everyone is a winner – everyone gets publicity and the moral capital that stems from being in the right, at least in the eyes of some – and where the front lines typically make use of trenches left behind by fighters of some other recent culture war. While superficially harmless, art wars follow the polarizing logic we know from terrorism and the war on terror (or rather, from their present-day seamless fusion where the one can hardly be told from the other).[10]

What is central – if you will, shocking – about *Piss Christ* lies in the artist's combination of the holy with excrement, a traditional object of devotion with an object of disgust. Serrano is consciously playing around with American and Catholic kitsch, here as well as in his other works. Yet his main objective is not necessarily (only) to shock the bourgeois. It is not easy to form a full idea of his intentions. But we may perhaps see Serrano as revitalizing a religious message that *ought* to shock us every time we enter a church. God as a torture victim – why do we not recognize this in the familiar shape of the crucifix? Is it because we have grown used to it or because of an inner resistance to the sight that meets us? That very message made Christianity so alien, unintelligible, impossible, unacceptable to the world of classical antiquity: in the words of the poet Andrew Hudgins, 'the whole irreducible point of faith,/ God thrown in human waste, submerged and shining'.Is it possible to admit that:

> He peed, ejaculated, shat, wept, bled –
> bled under Pontius Pilate, and I assume
> the mutilated god, the criminal,
> humiliated god, voided himself
> on the cross and blood and urine smeared his legs.[11]

By his choice of material and motif, Serrano also subscribes to a philosophical and literary discourse that should be thoroughly conventional and familiar to us by now. The fact that a work of art follows a convention is neither here nor there in itself. The convention has nevertheless become so convenient that an art critic has described her memories of the art of the 1980s and '90s as 'more or less a continuous flirt with the disgusting and terrifying, the abject'.[12] A flirt: it was not a case of introducing faecal matter as a new material among others in artistic use (urine has of course a long history of its own as a dyeing agent). The aim was not to neutralize 'the abject' but to keep its repulsive effect and to use it, the underlying idea being that our reaction to the abject *reveals* something important about us.

Resistance to square thinking

The instinctive and artistic defence of dirt was not an isolated phenomenon: it went hand in hand with theoretical ideas critical of the modernist cult of purity, rationality, hygiene, air and light. The critical trend shows no signs of abating and the symbiosis of art and theoretical approaches is now firmly established.[13] The dirty is now real life, the clean is plastic, whereas our longing for purity stands out as fear of life itself in its full messy detail, according to the principle 'whatever lives also soils, and all that cleans kills.'[14]

Some of the dystopian literature of the mid-twentieth century – such as Aldous Huxley's *Brave New World* – already takes issue with modernist pipe dreams. The story is set in a future when the clinically frictionless society is nearing completion. Those who live outside civilization are located in a hostile desert, which appears a threat but also has a strange appeal to more complex and hence more vulnerable souls in the midst of civilization. The moral lesson is that we can never create the perfect society unless we give up on something even more valuable: authenticity, which can only be preserved through the recognition of life's complexities and ambiguities.

At the theoretical level, aversion to modernism implies scepticism towards rationality. This of course makes it difficult to try to *refute* such scepticism with the help of established academic tools. There is no unity about the rules of the game. Romanticism about dirt is in itself an academic product, but when an *academic* lashes out against academia she will get the best of both worlds by playing simultaneously the insider and the outsider.[15] The pattern of rhetorical frontlines reminds us of the art wars. On the losing, conservative side are the defenders of conventional square thinking. On the winning, progressive side stands the critical thinker who has freed herself of illusions and compulsive disorders rooted in the common man's fear of the stranger, of the Other.

Dirt as emancipation

Fears of dirt and contagion have repeatedly been harnessed for political use. Research has highlighted direct continuities between the hygienic campaigns of the early twentieth century and contemporaneous campaigns for racial purity, with the aim of cleansing the national body politic of disturbing elements. Political philosopher Martha Nussbaum has pointed to the role of ideas of purity in the oppression of women and sexual minorities, historian Klaus Theweleit has studied proto-Nazi fantasies of sexual, ideological and racial purity while, even more alarmingly, sociologist Zygmunt Bauman has elaborated on connections between cleanliness and ethnic cleansing.[16]

No one should be surprised to find various typically human emotions and attitudes put to evil use. One may ask if it is even possible to find some human trait that is quite immune to misuse. For instance, laughter and jokes may foster feelings of togetherness but also of hostility. And who can count all those who put others to suffer at the stake in the name of love and virtue? We should therefore investigate the widely spread suggestion that ideas of dirt and purity not only *can* be misused but that the connection between cleanliness and oppression is much more intimate.

According to Nussbaum, our concern for cleanliness, at least as it has developed in present Western culture, represents a tendency *inherently* hostile to life. In her essay "'The Secret Sewers of Vice": Disgust, Bodies, and the Law' Nussbaum presents an analysis of disgust.[17] She obviously wants her analysis to be applicable to cleanliness more generally, because on the whole she implies that our relation to dirt is informed by feelings of disgust.[18] Her paper is interesting not least because, even though she hails from the English-speaking analytical tradition and stays generally close to the current mainstream of North American political philosophy, she takes up ideas quite similar to ones expressed in the European Continental debate on abjection. One strand of Nussbaum's essay consists of criticism of the use of 'disgust' as an argument in legal theory, especially by theorists and judges with conservative leanings. Her political diagnosis, which is perhaps independent of her general analysis of disgust, need not detain us here. The more interesting idea for the present purpose is Nussbaum's association of our present preoccupation with cleanliness with a general refusal to accept the fact of our embodied animal nature.[19]

In her analysis of disgust as an emotion, Nussbaum is partly drawing on William Miller's book *The Anatomy of Disgust* (1997), and partly on experimental research by the psychologist Paul Rozin.[20] She describes disgust mainly as a sort of resistance against the perceived invasion of the body by contaminating substances. It involves the defence of the subject's bodily integrity against the threat of contamination or absorption.[21] Disgust is, however, not a purely physiological reaction: it is based on the subject's *judgements* of the identity of the rejected substance and thus, unlike the feeling of distaste or the sense of danger, disgust is motivated by 'ideational factors'. Nussbaum claims moreover that this defence of bodily integrity is *symbolic*. 'The ideational content of disgust is that the self will become base or contaminated by ingestion of the substance that is viewed as offensive.'[22]

Nussbaum argues, in other words, that our feelings of disgust are in important cases based on associations that should really strike us as false and irrational. Disgust is triggered by a kind of implicit and unacknowledged belief in 'sympathetic magic': the idea that by touching, objects – including our bodies and, by extension, our persons – *become* like the objects touched.[23] Disgust is our way of mentally shielding ourselves against the fact that we are embodied beings subject to decay. 'In all societies . . . disgust expresses a refusal to ingest and thus be contaminated by a potent reminder of one's own mortality and animality.'[24] These associations are particularly sinister because they hold the potential of singling out unwanted human groups as less than human. Moreover, Nussbaum holds that they are also misogynic since women are traditionally, more so than men, associated with the body.[25] The problematic role of disgust in society can be put aright only through 'a re-creation of our entire relationship to the bodily'. Quoting Walt Whitman, Nussbaum concludes that

> The job of the poet of democracy therefore becomes that of singing 'the body electric,' establishing that the locus of common human need and aspiration is fundamentally acceptable and pleasing.[26]

A laudable goal, no doubt – although one might wonder whether celebration of the body would have to translate to a 'celebration' of all of its fluids.

What is Nussbaum's argument for the claim that reactions of disgust are our way of fending off our animal nature? According to Nussbaum, it has been 'confirmed experimentally that "all disgust objects are animals or animal products," or objects that have had contact with animals or animal products – a major source being contact with "people who are disliked or viewed as unsavory".'[27] Nussbaum is surely right in pointing out that many of the substances we tend to describe as disgusting are animal products.[28] On the other hand, this would not be surprising, considering the fact that disgust is very typically connected with eating; and many foodstuffs are animal products.[29] Moreover, practically *everything* in our environment will be 'animal' in the extremely wide sense that Nussbaum allows: either having animal origin, having 'had contact with animals or animal products', or somehow *reminding* us of animals – especially if 'people who are disliked' are also to count as *animal*. A question that now would arise is why we are not disgusted simply all the time.

In addition to questions of detail, we should ask whether it is meaningful in the first place to compose a list of 'disgusting things' as such, quite regardless of the situation. Is it really possible to identify a substance that we would just always describe as disgusting – always and everywhere?[30] Conversely, is it possible to find something that no one would *ever* feel to be disgusting? Nussbaum also apparently takes it to be a matter of course that our dominant reaction to dirt is that of disgust. Perhaps I need here to make the commonplace observation that disgust, *pace* many writers addressing the topic, is by no means our only possible reaction to dirt; it is hardly even the most frequent one. For instance, our ordinary cleaning efforts are hardly dominated by a constant sense of disgust.

Whatever else we may think of Nussbaum's analysis of disgust, it certainly illustrates the theoretical debate of the last decades on the topic of dirt and excreta. The dominating trend can be described as one of 'craving for generality' and a 'contemptuous attitude towards the particular case'.[31] In addition, there is a certain predilection, whenever possible, for shocking descriptions that supposedly are representative of the field of pollution and abjection in its entirety. This perhaps does not indicate interest in the concepts of dirty and clean so much as a need of powerful metaphors in general debates on culture and society.

As a sometimes negligent householder, but still proud of my intellectual credentials, I am naturally soothed by the idea that exaggerated cleanliness is not next to godliness but to fascism and xenophobia, plus any number of other convenient phobias. Yet in reading the defences of dirt published in the last couple of decades, and considering in particular against what and *whom* dirt has been defended, I cannot help seeing the debate as just one more round in the Achilles-and-tortoise game of symbolic class struggle. The new middle class, struggling to forget its working-class roots, has now secured the trappings of urban respectability. In response, *real* intellectuals, anxious to keep their distance from the newcomers, no longer feel like admitting in public that they, too, like to have it nice and clean around them. The Swedish journalist Per Svensson sums it up:

A neglected and dusty home may confirm that here live charming and creative artistic types, or extremely successful and busy professionals who have more important things to worry about than keeping it clean in every corner. Dust-heaps in corners may also be seen as cute pets in a family that sets store on precisely the Family and Being with the Children and What Is Valuable in Life, not on shining hardwood floors. A sparkling clean home may, then, invite suspicion; it may hint of Angst, square thinking, narrow-mindedness, deep-frozen emotional life, closet sadism and inability to orgasm.[32]

Art and rubbish

But is there not enough evidence to show that the difference between clean and dirty may turn out to be simply a convention with no solid base in reality? Perhaps 'the man on the street' simply has naive ideas of what stuff everyday life is made of? Consider a story that, in October 2001, made it to the headlines, together with Osama bin Laden and V. S. Naipaul:

Cleaner clears up Hirst's ashtray art

It is often said that modern art is rubbish, but never did it ring as true as when an art gallery cleaner binned a work by Damien Hirst because he thought the installation was exactly that – leftover rubbish. Emmanuel Asare thought the piles of full ashtrays, half-filled coffee cups, empty beer bottles and newspapers strewn across the gallery were the remnants of a party in the west London gallery. Although that is what it was, this rubbish had been arranged by Hirst into an impromptu installation, which increased its value by thousands . . . 'As soon as I clapped eyes on it I sighed because there was so much mess. I didn't think for a second that it was a work of art – it didn't look much like art to me.' . . . Staff were dispatched to find the binbags in the rubbish, and salvaged the various objects, which they used to reconstruct the installation from photographs taken earlier. Hirst, 35, said the piles of junk represented an artist's studio and said the mistake was 'fantastic. Very funny.' Charles Thomson, co-founder of the Stuckist art movement, which favours the traditional skills of drawing and painting, praised Mr Asare's action. 'The cleaner obviously ought to be promoted to an art critic of a national newspaper. He clearly has a fine critical eye' . . . he said.[33]

The first reaction by the theoretically sophisticated reader might be, 'Told you so.' The news report seems to confirm the completely subjective and conventional character of artistic appreciation, and by the same token, the arbitrariness of classifying an object as dirt or rubbish.

But let us be open-minded also about our presumptions of open-mindedness. Hirst was hardly intent on inviting disinterested, purely aesthetic reactions. Whatever power may lie in his installation is completely dependent on the ambiguity which the onlooker is expected to recognize and solve: the installation is art *and* rubbish *at once*, which is why it needs to be recognizable (also) as precisely rubbish. This implies in fact that what counts as 'rubbish' is *not* purely conventional. Hirst's *artwork* acquires its essential artistic effect from the fact that the identities of objects are not up to us to decide: it consists of rubbish *objectively*, independently of the observer.

The grammar of dirty and clean: a statement of mission

In philosophy, to ask 'What is dirt?' is to inquire about the *concept of* dirt. To analyse the concept is to ask what is *meant by* 'dirt' and related expressions as they are used in various life situations. This is not to look for a definition of any kind but rather to produce what may be called philosophical grammar: a perspicuous presentation of the difference that the concept makes to us – including both the problems that it solves for us and the new ones it creates. Such descriptions of grammar are inscribed in historical times and places, which is why they need to be constantly rewritten and reconsidered. Every now and then, the philosophical task also requires us to take account of foreign cultures and of our own past, but the central task remains the one of spelling out the meaning of 'dirt' and 'dirty' for us – current members of Western industrialized societies. For reasons of principle, cultural variation cannot demonstrate that our current practices somehow really and at bottom amount to something exotic and quite different from what we have, until now, *believed* they are – just as little as the discovery of *similarities* between our practices and those of 'Farawaystan' would confirm the correctness of our own ideas.[34] We need comparisons between dirt and various related concepts, but the bottom line is that dirt is not identical to any of its siblings and cousins. The discussion of the extent to which dirt resembles other categories or differs from them is, however, important because it helps us locate it on a conceptual map. What I chiefly have in mind is practical cleanliness, not metaphorical, ritual or religious purity, even though the demarcation between the practical and the symbolic must itself be a matter of reflection.

The recent resurgence of theoretical and artistic attention to purity and pollution perhaps just marks a healthy return to questions artificially left aside for a period of Western cultural history. On the other hand, it may also indicate that cleanliness practices are not quite as self-evident to us as they once were. In modern societies marked by professionalism and division of labour, our relations to everyday material objects often betray a sense of alienation, of loss of control. We know how to throw things away but no longer how to clean and mend.

TWO

A Brief History of Dirt in Philosophy

The Greeks of old

The philosophy of dirt is approximately the same age as Western science and philosophy in general – except they were not 'Western' in the beginning, but should be called Levantine if we insist on imposing a geographical specification. When we now chart the development of this work, the result must be nothing less than a history of philosophy *sub specie sordis* (from the point of view of dirt).[1] For obvious reasons, this account must be both cursory and highly selective, a main criterion being relevance from a modern point of view. We find that the problem of dirt has been omnipresent in philosophy, as it has been involved in all its major upheavals and developments. Insofar as the nature of reality – or more properly, the nature of our *concepts of* reality[2] – has been a concern for philosophy, its views will in part have been formulated via different positions vis-à-vis those aspects of physical reality that strike the philosopher as particularly problematic.

The *Fragments* of Heraclitus, from the sixth to fifth centuries BCE, mark the beginning of the philosophical discourse on soiling. Heraclitus' work does not survive in its entirety, but informed reconstructions of his philosophy are possible. Several of the extant fragments bear witness to an apparently fully developed view on the clean and the dirty. It appears that the Ionian philosopher repeatedly made use of ideas of dirt and impurity in arguments in support of a kind of philosophical relativism in the making. He wonders at the religious rites of his time – including

animal sacrifice where blood simultaneously appears as both
defilement and purification:

> Tainted with blood they purify themselves in a different
> way as if someone who stepped into mud were cleansed
> with mud. But any human who claimed that the person
> was doing that would be considered insane. And they pray
> to these statues, as if someone, who knew nothing of what
> gods or heroes are like, were to converse with the houses.[3]

Heraclitus described the expiatory rite as a case of washing away
blood with blood, a point immediately intelligible to his con-
temporaries. The Greek word μίασμα (*miasma*) was applied to
both soiling (especially blood stains) and moral guilt. The concept
was later rendered in Latin as *piaculum*, a word that means both
'expiatory rite, atonement' and 'sin', the crime that *requires* the
sin-offering. This may be further compared with Greek μίαστωρ
(*miastōr*), which stands both for the person guilty of sin and the
one whose duty it is to exact vengeance. Both exist in a state of
emergency or otherness: the one because of a crime committed and
the other through the revenge still not carried out. We are, in other
words, now dealing with a tradition which, since time immemorial,
associates moral guilt with dirt and smell. Its earliest documents
are almost as old as the art of writing. The Papyrus of Ani, a copy
of *The Egyptian Book of the Dead* (1500–1400 BCE), describes the
perilous journey of the soul to Ialu, the abode of the blessed.
During this journey the soul needs to purify itself, uttering a
prayer with the words: 'May the *shenit* [a class of divine beings]
not cause my name to stink, and may not lies be spoken against
me in the presence of the god.'[4] And further in another place:
'Deliver thou [me] from the great god who carrieth away souls,
and who devoureth filth and eateth dirt, the guardian of the
darkness [who himself liveth] in the light. They who are in misery
fear him.'[5]

In manuscripts, the Eater of Dirt is depicted as a horrifying creature with a crocodile face. A late descendant of this animal is sometimes found in medieval and Baroque Christian art, still in his old habit of devouring sinners in Hell.

But now returning to Heraclitus: from a modern point of view it is easy to interpret his critique of priests who wash away blood with blood and who talk with statues as an ironic comment on un-enlightened practices and superstition. However, the ironic edge is blunted as soon as we realize that Heraclitus wants to be relativist about the very concept of impurity. In fact animals *are* perfectly able to wash themselves in dirt: 'Swine wash in the mire, and barn-yard fowls in dust.'[6] Dirt is something quite different for men and animals: 'The sea is the purest and the impurest water. Fish can drink it, and it is good for them; to men it is undrinkable and destructive.'[7]

If, then, those who participate in religious ceremonies *appear* just as crazy as someone who talks with houses or 'delight[s] in the mire',[8] this only goes to show the inadequacy of human reason. The expiatory rite can be perceived in two ways: in a divine and religious way, where we indeed *do* wash away blood with blood, and in a secular human way where it makes no sense to talk with stones and buildings.[9] This reading of Heraclitus presents him as making a relativist point, something highlighted especially if we go along with Catherine (Rowett) Osborne's translation of Heraclitus' opening words on the expiatory rite: 'They purify themselves in a different way,' as opposed to an earlier reading, 'They vainly purify themselves.'[10] Just as human beings and animals see the world differently, so do human beings and gods, for 'the human way has no sense, but the divine way does'.[11] No wonder 'Heraclitus has considered human opinions to be children's toys.'[12]

And if Heraclitus indeed points out that 'corpses are more fit to be cast out than dung',[13] to be sure this runs against ordinary thinking – but it just goes to show that most of us walk through life as in a dream, where 'the most perfect of all worlds is just a dung-heap.'[14] We can read Heraclitus as saying that various human and animal life forms each follow their own logic. These life forms are relative, context-dependent, both correct and incorrect depending on how you look at them. But in addition to the earthly perspectives of human beings and animals there seems to be one more perspective: that of the gods. The latter may also be available 'to men who are entirely purified, which . . . rarely happens to one man, or to a certain easily to be numbered few of mankind'.[15] From the divine perspective, apparently the concepts of dirty and clean lose their meanings altogether: 'To a god all things are fair and good and right, but men hold some things wrong and some right.'[16]

Summing up, and with due caution owing to the fragmentary nature of the sources, the first appearance of dirt over the philosophical horizon appears in many ways to be a negative affair. For Heraclitus, ideas of dirt are above all a symptom of the limitations of human understanding. As long as we keep within the bounds of the human and mortal, Heraclitus does not seem to imagine an internal ranking of perspectives: all mortal beings fall pitifully short of the truth – the true view which is enjoyed by gods but seldom if ever attained by humans. On the other hand, all different human and animal perspectives express some relative truth. Our notions of dirt are not more, but also no *less* true than, for instance, the thinking of animals.

Forms of formlessness

Slightly more than a hundred years later, Plato takes up some of the threads left by Heraclitus. Like his predecessor he describes ordinary thinking as mere opinion (*doxa*), relative and changeable, contrasting it with true knowledge (*epistēmē*). In contrast with Heraclitus, however, Plato presents the pursuit of true knowledge as a difficult but yet *possible* human undertaking. Its basis lies in reason and intuition, expressed in philosophy and mathematics, two activities that share some of the qualities Heraclitus ascribed to the Divine.

The proper objects of real knowledge are the *Forms*, also, especially in older translations, known as (Platonic) Ideas. Forms can be defined as models or prototypes. They are the essences or first principles of the things that we, in everyday life, tend to *call* reality, and our entire understanding of reality is only made possible by Forms. It is easiest to see what Plato is after if we think of his favoured example, the role of geometry in human life. No one has ever had the experience of a perfect circle: perfect circles do not exist in our environment. And no one has seen a circle that is *only* circle, only geometrical shape: every circle we have experienced has been at the same time a coloured surface circumscribed by lines, for instance drawn in pencil, coal, ink or a stick in the sand. Nevertheless, the real circle, the Form of the circle, exists. It 'exists' because it is necessary for our thinking and knowledge: we recognize existing approximations of the circular form as such only because we understand them in relation to the proper geometrical figure. The Form is also the *origin* of all circular drawings in existence, because we can *try to* draw a circle only insofar as we have this understanding. Last but not least, we understand deviations from the standard as *imperfections* because we implicitly compare the circle we draw with the Form. Generalizing from this: rational thinking about reality is possible only insofar as things of reality conform to Forms. Conversely, we gain our knowledge of the Forms precisely by extrapolating from the experiences we do have in an imperfectly designed world.

What are the implications of this to ideas of dirt? This is exactly the question that Plato takes up in his dialogue *Parmenides*, ostensibly a discussion between Socrates and the philosopher Parmenides. Socrates, then a young man, has just voiced his conviction that all things have Forms. Parmenides then asks him whether he thinks this also holds true of 'things of which the mention may provoke a smile' – 'such things as hair, mud, dirt, or anything else which is vile and paltry'. Does Dirt have a Form? The rub is that both 'yes' and 'no' would seem to lead to absurdity. Let me now enlarge on this issue.

We are now feeling the main pulse of antiquity. Its world view was essentially teleological. A thing was defined in terms of its 'point', its goal or *telos*. To grasp the essence of a thing was, among other things, to be able to tell good from bad instances of the thing. Consider a knife. The definition of a knife is primarily that of a *good* knife, one that can be used for cutting purposes – and more precisely for cutting wood, hair or butter. On the whole, Greeks liked to think of physical objects along the lines of tools, functional artefacts; mainly not in analogy with natural objects like stones or as undefined 'matter'. On this question, Martin Heidegger remarks, 'The Greeks had an appropriate term for 'Things': πράγματα [*prágmata*] – that is to say, that which one has to do with in one's concernful dealings (πρᾶξις) [*prâxis*].'[17] A thing had its own life, existence, teleology: a knife, a pencil, an apple tree, an egg are defined in terms of their potentialities for cutting, writing, bearing fruit and hatching a chicken. In the light of this understanding of the nature of 'things', it is both possible and imperative to ask *to what extent* an individual thing lives up to its Form or essence.

At this point, the existence of soiling creates a difficulty. If everything has a Form in the Platonic sense, this should also be true of soiling, as well as of other phenomena classified as defects. The Forms were supposed to be the essence or perfection of the things they were Forms of. But things 'vile and paltry' are defined in terms of falling short of the ideal. What would the Form of *that* be? The Form of not having a Form, the perfect imperfection? In his discussion with Parmenides, Socrates initially and rather pathetically denies that such Forms can be admitted:

> Certainly not, said Socrates; visible things like these are such as they appear to us, and I am afraid that there would be an absurdity in assuming any idea [*viz*. Form] of them,

although I sometimes get disturbed, and begin to think that there is nothing without [a Form]; but then again, when I have taken up this position, I run away, because I am afraid that I may fall into a bottomless pit of nonsense, and perish; and so I return to the [Forms] of which I was just now speaking [identity, unity, plurality, the Right, etc.], and occupy myself with them.[18]

Later interpreters have struggled to find a tenable position with regard to Plato's views on 'the other' – *héteron* (ἕτερον), the negative, opposing pole of a given concept that belongs to a pair of opposites. Is, for instance, the ugly merely the absence of the beautiful? Do evil and injustice exist as phenomena in their own right or do they simply consist in the absence of goodness and justice? The latter interpretation was dominant since at least St Augustine, who of course was drawing on the neo-Platonic tradition and not only on Plato's own writings. In modern debate, interpreters leaning on *The Sophist* and *The Republic*[19] have argued that Plato may well have counted on Forms of 'the other'. But it is quite possible that Plato had no definite standpoint.[20] After all, he had no obligation to have an answer to *every* issue that future readers might want to question him about. We do find, however, that he was aware of the need of unprejudiced thinking and of questioning one's pet theories. Here is Parmenides' reply to Socrates as Plato imagines it:

Yes, Socrates, said Parmenides; that is because you are still young; the time will come, if I am not mistaken, when philosophy will have a firmer grasp of you, and then you will not despise even the meanest things; at your age, you are too much disposed to regard the opinions of men.[21]

In the history of ancient philosophy, the philosophy of Aristotle is often contrasted against that of Plato, his teacher. Aristotle was certainly more open to empirical research, especially in biology.

He – or probably, some student of his – was not above writing a short book on 'Problems Connected with Unpleasant Smells' (Book XIII of *Problemata Physica*),[22] among other things dealing with questions such as:

- Why do unpleasant odours seem not to smell to those who have eaten?
- Why do all things smell more when in motion?
- Why is the smell of the breath heavier and more unpleasant in the deformed and stooping?[23]

The questions are addressed within the general framework of the medical theory of the times, focusing on the distribution of various elements, like humidity, in different bodies. Aristotle, furthermore, pays attention to the concept of *mutilation* or *damage* in his *Metaphysics* and he discusses biological deformations in his book on the development of animals.[24]

However, despite Aristotle's interest in empirical research, which marks him off from Plato, and despite their disagreements about the status of the Forms, what unites the two thinkers is their shared belief in essences; the idea of the Form as expressing the real essence of objects. The legacy of the Greeks in general and of Plato in particular apparently includes an idea of different *degrees of reality* pertaining to objects. Soiling and damage imply that the reality of the object is in some sense diminished, as the object is brought further away from its essence. In this context, the idea of studying nature is not separable from the conception of the natural as a normative concept. Not everything that exists is equally natural. Physical reality itself contains degrees of reality – associated with order and the good – and unreality, associated with chaos and evil. The more one identifies 'reality' with the true and the good (and the more capitalized one wants these words to be) the more problematic is the status of dirt as part of reality.

Alchemy and the problem of perishability

Reflections on the general theme of decay are an integral part of Christian theology. Starting with St Paul, decay is treated as part of the problem of theodicy. In the material world, things characteristically fall short of their inherent teleologies in all kinds of ways, but how can this be the case if they are created by God who is love?

The physical perishability of the created environment, including our own bodies, has a very old religious explanation: material decay originates in man's Fall from God or the gods, driving a wedge between God and the world. This tradition assumes a direct correspondence between the fate of humankind and that of material reality. Our own steadily advancing moral decay is mirrored in nature. In *Works and Days*, Hesiod (end of 8th century BCE) describes the earlier ages of humankind as a succession where the constantly declining quality of life correlates with the decline of morals and the debasement of metal value. After the Golden Age come the Silver, Bronze and finally Iron Age.[25] Each successive human race is destroyed because of its own trespasses. The present men of iron are the worst, of whom Hesiod says, 'I wish I were not of this race.'[26] When the last traces of decency are gone, this final breed of men will also be wiped off the face of the earth.

In *Epistle to the Romans* St Paul draws our attention specifically to the parallel between the Fall of Adam and natural decay: just as all humans are sinners, nature, like all flesh, is slave to sin. Because of sin, physical decay was introduced. Like humans, nature is yearning for redemption:

> For the creation waits with eager longing for the revealing of the children of God; for the creation was subjected to futility, not of its own will but by the will of the one who subjected it, in hope that the creation itself will be set free from its bondage to decay and will obtain the freedom of the glory of the children of God. We know that the whole

creation has been groaning in labor pains until now; and not only the creation, but we ourselves, who have the first fruits of the Spirit, groan inwardly while we wait for adoption, the redemption of our bodies.[27]

The shared condition of perishability and the shared hope one day to overcome it creates a bond between man and creation. But the human individual, unlike nature, can find the way to redemption through moral and religious rebirth.

Mortality as such was introduced to the world through the Fall of man. The generally agreed medieval theory was, furthermore, that the processes of decay were accelerating with time. This had particularly been the case in the period after the Flood, which saw both an increase of polluted matter and the weakening of nature's nourishing and remedial powers enshrined in plants, fruit and seeds. To be sure, God had distributed medicinal and life-prolonging herbs into nature but they alone could not compensate for the loss of a pristine milieu. In consequence, the expected human life span had decreased dramatically. We can only count on a few decades of life while Adam's immediate descendants lived for nearly a thousand years.[28]

These ideas became the ideological starting point for the tradition of alchemy. Its theological justification was found in St Paul, who believed that the road to salvation was laid out not only for human beings but for animals and even inorganic nature.[29] The individual's personal development and aspirations toward purity were exactly mirrored in natural processes of maturation. Seeds would become trees and fruit would grow ripe on trees. Metals would mutate into other metals through decay or maturation; gold would develop in the earth's womb. Not everything would turn into gold, just as vices would not be mutated into virtues, so one needed to intensify the good tendencies in metals and dismiss materials that would not accompany them to salvation – dregs, refuse, slags, materials that corresponded to sin in human life. Martin Luther, who was generally appreciative of St Paul, took up the idea in his *Table Talk* (1566):

> The science of alchymy I like very well, and, indeed, 'tis the philosophy of the ancients. I like it not only for the profits it brings in melting metals, in decocting, preparing, extracting, and distilling herbs, roots; I like it also for the sake of the allegory and secret signification, which is exceedingly fine, touching the resurrection of the dead at the last day. For, as in a furnace the fire extracts and separates from a substance the other portions, and carries upward the spirit, the life, the sap, the strength, while the unclean matter, the dregs, remain at the bottom, like a dead and worthless carcass; even so God, at the day of judgement, will separate all things through fire, the righteous from the ungodly. The Christians and righteous shall ascend upward into heaven, and there live everlastingly, but the wicked and the ungodly, as the dross and filth, shall remain in hell, and there be damned.[30]

Alchemy was thus connected with the idea that the human soul and nature were intertwined elements of an undivided creation. Man would help both himself and the pure elements of creation to salvation. Physical reality was destined one day to be completely purified and glorified; this is a recurring motif in the Old and New Testaments. Isaiah, accusing his people of moral decline, tells them, 'Your silver has become dross,' but God, coming in His wrath, 'will smelt away your dross as with lye and remove all your alloy'.[31] To Malachi, God appears like the fire of the goldsmith or the lye of the washer, which will 'purify the descendants of Levi and refine them like gold and silver, until they present offerings to the Lord in righteousness'.[32] Finally, in the Revelation, heavenly Jerusalem will come descending from the heaven, but this rebuilt version is entirely composed of purified, 'eternal' materials:

The wall is built of jasper, while the city is pure gold, clear
as glass. The foundations of the wall of the city are adorned
with every jewel; the first was jasper, the second sapphire,
the third agate, the fourth emerald, the fifth onyx, the sixth
carnelian, the seventh chrysolite, the eighth beryl, the ninth
topaz, the tenth chrysoprase, the eleventh jacinth, the twelfth
amethyst. And the twelve gates are twelve pearls, each of
the gates is a single pearl, and the street of the city is pure
gold, transparent as glass.[33]

Modern chemistry is far removed from the kind of vitalist
view of inorganic nature taken for granted by its alchemistic predecessor, a fact that we must view with due appreciation.[34] On the
other hand we should not exaggerate the contrast between alchemy
and our present understanding of reality. We certainly should not
become alchemists again, but we might at least recognize alchemy
as an enlarging mirror that helps us understand our natural attitudes. In important ways it is merely a hermetic outgrowth from
a self-evident and probably necessary perspective on the natural
world. Just consider the fact that we still wait for fruit to grow ripe
and still throw away spoiled produce. Natural processes always
and everywhere include the undoing of earlier structures and the
development of new ones – consider the growth of mould on food.
The key to understanding the idea of decay does not, however, lie
in the organic processes as such but in the teleological distinction
between processes that are in harmony with the object's *telos* (for
example, the ripening of French cheese) and processes that are not.

Alchemy should also give us a better perspective on the current
debate on 'abjection'. In the academic debate today, our relation
to dirt is often presented as a kind of negative and Angst-ridden
attitude towards natural processes. Alchemy, in contrast, presents
the human relationship to physical nature in terms of guardianship
and care. To fight against soiling is to protect and nourish natural
tendencies towards perfection both in nature and in ourselves.

The new science

Giovanni Pico, Count Mirandola (1463–1494), was a member of the Platonic Academy of Florence, a freshly created (and short-lived) learned society with aspirations to re-create what was best in the philosophy of the ancients. Pico della Mirandola's speech *Oration on the Dignity of Man* is often cited as the opening words of Florentine Renaissance, the dawn of modern man waking to the consciousness of his own worth.[35] Conveniently enough, the most frequently quoted passages come right at the beginning – a veritable hymn of praise to the human being and the human limitless power of free development.

A critical reader will find, however, that the work as a whole is a motley collection of ideas – indicating that Renaissance Italy had more strings to its bow than the bloodless marble beauty that later generations popularly associate with it. We must remember that alchemy, too, was more of a Renaissance movement than a medieval remnant – just like the witch hunts, which reached their peak in the seventeenth century. Pico's speech connects with the re-emergence of Platonic ideas which also inspired the development of alchemy. Pico wants to see both natural science and the Holy Scriptures in the light of neo-Platonism. Man can both ascend to the level of angels and descend to the level of animals. As in alchemy, the almost limitless existential freedom of the human being is set in a context of *preordained* levels of moral and natural creation. Purification is the overarching symbol of human progress: we must 'purify our souls' with the help of rational thinking, 'thus washing away, so to speak, the filth of ignorance and vice,'[36] and wash our dirty hands and feet 'in moral philosophy as in a living stream.'[37]

Some of Pico's ideas appear today as blind alleys (such as his references to the occult wisdom of Hermes Trismegistos and the Chaldaeans[38]) while others look like anticipations of future triumphs of science. Thus he speaks of 'a new method of philosophizing on the basis of numbers'. This method, he tells us, 'is, in fact, very old'.[39] Here he appeals to both well-known and more obscure predecessors, including Pythagoras and Plato, but also Homer and the less well-known figures of Zamolxis and Zoroaster the son of Oromasius.[40] A hundred years later, Galileo took up this strand when he argued that the Book of Nature was *scritta in lingua matematica*, 'written in the language of mathematics'.[41] Similarly, Kepler's laws of the movements of the celestial bodies were developed as a direct continuation of the Pythagorean doctrine of mathematical harmony in nature.

The Renaissance return to Platonism and the dismissal of Aristotle created the conditions for the growth of experimental science. This may appear paradoxical because, of the two thinkers, Aristotle had been the one to emphasize the need of facts and observation. It is, however, surprising only unless we keep in mind that 'observation' for Aristotle was something quite different from the mathematically informed research programmes that started to dominate Western science. Modern science does not simply sit down and wait for experiences to happen but *creates* them in carefully organized – and sometimes completely 'unnatural' – experimental settings. Thus the growing irrelevance of Aristotle was due to the fact that he stayed too close to nature, not that he strayed away from it. The modern Book of Nature is a book of accounts, not a travel diary.

By making an appeal to ancient philosophical authority, the fledgling modern science secured the right to disregard immediate experience. Immediate experience now came across as *constitutively unable* to capture the nature of reality. This was, in particular, expressed in the doctrine of primary and secondary qualities.

Primary and secondary qualities

Seventeenth-century natural philosophy developed a strategy for assimilating the new scientific results, whereby two elements were distinguished. The one element, nature 'out there' as it is *in itself* regardless of anyone who happens to observe it, was isolated from the rest, a subjective element which was the contribution of the human perceptual faculties. This approach was expressed in the doctrine of primary and secondary qualities. The main idea was already formulated by the ancient Atomists and found a supporter in Galileo, but its most influential formulation was included in John Locke's *Essay Concerning Human Understanding* in 1690. Locke, who had for a time worked as an assistant in Robert Boyle's chemical laboratory, wanted to deal a final blow to the medieval Aristotelian doctrine of 'real accidents' and instead to propagate the 'corpuscular hypothesis' about the structure of material reality.

Primary qualities – according to Locke, 'solidity, extension, figure, motion or rest, and number' – 'really exist in the bodies themselves'.[42] Secondary qualities such as colour, sound, taste, odour and temperature are, instead, 'in truth nothing in the objects themselves' but only ideas caused by the action of primary qualities on the sense organs.[43] For instance, the white colour and cold feel of a snowball are caused by the microscopic qualities and configurations of the corpuscles (that is, particles) it is made of. Their powers to create sensations in a human subject are similar to the power of an emetic in that their microscopic structure stimulates certain feelings in the body.[44] But feeling sick is not a quality of *the emetic* any more than pain is a quality of the knife that wounds my finger. Similarly, colour, sound, temperature, taste and odour merely consist in the powers of the object to stimulate psychological responses (sensations) in the human subject.[45]

On the whole, modern natural philosophy has remained true to Locke's approach, even though research now presents a more nuanced picture of the microscopic detail, and the list of plausible primary qualities is constantly developing.[46] Locke based his list on the idea that objective qualities of the physical world can be described in terms of spatial extension. Today, lists of possible primary qualities are no longer handed down to physicists by philosophers but the other way around – now including qualities like *spin*, which does not include spatial extension in its definition. The precise list as such is not, perhaps, of crucial philosophical interest, but the important point is that philosophers have now agreed to delegate the question of 'the ultimate constituents of the natural world' to *physicists*. Physics is now thought of as the authority on the 'natural world' while another, opposite realm of psychology and subjectivity is carved out for the humanities.

If dirt is described as the psychological effect of the qualities – primary and secondary – of objects on us, it might be classified as a 'tertiary' quality.[47] From the point of view of corpuscular or materialist natural philosophy, dirt holds no interest – except perhaps as an example of our confused mental habit of projecting subjective qualities into objects.

Dirt as a 'tertiary' quality

The idea that certain perceived qualities of the world are subjective follows naturally from the doctrine of primary and secondary qualities, but it got a new twist when Romantic historical consciousness started to question the idea that the human psyche is everywhere the same. Our experience of the world mirrors not only the general human condition but culturally specific circumstances. It is left to the anthropological disciplines to study the psychological, cultural and social mechanisms that assumedly give a subjective colouring to the physical world. The renewal of philosophical interest in soiling was connected with the development of anthropological research, starting in the late nineteenth century. In the general cultural consciousness of the time, anthropology was not only supposed to answer specific questions about various non-industrial cultures of the global South; research on 'savages' would clarify issues concerning the essence and destiny of man. Insofar as it is today possible to talk of a received philosophical view on dirt, it, too, is a result of this anthropological discourse.

The received theoretical view is expressed well in an essay by the ethnologist Jonas Frykman. It is the introductory discussion to a study of the ideas of cleanliness among Swedish peasants and bourgeois at the beginning of the twentieth century:

> Such feelings [of disgust and distaste] which we experience as natural and instinctive are in fact culturally determined to an extreme degree. The concepts of 'disgusting', 'dirty' and their close relatives are not qualities that exist in objects as such. We are the ones who ascribe the spittoon or the snot-rag the power to disgust. Disgust as a feeling quite certainly exists, but what we find distasteful is something we learn.[48]

Frykman, however, makes things a bit too easy for himself by assuming an unwarranted identity between 'dirty' and 'disgusting'. A reader with a feel for the language (both in the original Swedish and in my translation) might also react to Frykman's assurance that 'the *concepts of* disgusting and dirty are not '*qualities* that exist *in objects* as such'. Quite apart from the fact that 'concepts' are, anyway, not qualities, there is something strange about the implied idea that qualities, in order to count as real, must exist 'in' objects. Objects indeed have qualities, but qualities do not exist inside them like cherries in a cake; which is why we say a snowball is round and a stone is hard, but typically not that roundness exists in the snowball and hardness in the stone. And what *is* round – that is also something 'we learn', presumably because we live in a culture where the concept of 'round' is used.

It is not easy to pin down the allegedly widespread popular confusion that Frykman claims to have identified and disarmed. We typically motivate disgust by pointing to something *disgusting* about the object in question, not by saying that disgust exists *in* it. The rather awkward phrase 'qualities that exist in objects' in Frykman's description is in fact carried over from Locke's original

Essay. Locke had wanted to voice his disagreement with the medieval doctrine of real accidents. That old theory had presupposed that certain qualities would be understood along the line of something existing in the object – say, a warm or caloric substance would explain the presence of warmth. Frykman's strange phrasing is a last trace of Locke's polemic against a physical theory that is now more or less defunct.

In all events we should note a rather massive consensus in contemporary theoretical thinking with regard to dirt: dirt is not really dirt but something else. It seems to me that reductionist views of this kind are accepted rather too easily.

THREE

Dirty and Clean: Main Distinctions

> We must look for intentions of nature in things which
> retain their nature, and not in things which are corrupted.
>
> Aristotle, *Politics*[1]

'Dirty' and 'dirt'

We are familiar with the word, but when do we use it and for what purposes? A quick first glance indicates that 'dirty' is a word typically applied to objects, substances, places and living beings or their parts. Also a person's way of life and habits may be described as dirty, as well as various ideas, intentions and other features of his or her moral life. In any case it is possible to say that 'dirt' and 'dirty' originally belong to descriptions of material objects, from which other usages historically seem to be derived. English 'dirt' probably comes from Old Norse *drit*, 'excrement'.[2] In this early use, the word stood for a specifiable substance. A rather similar usage still exists as a special case, when 'dirt' is employed to mean a kind of earth, as in 'road dirt' and 'dirt pie', or as the non-productive soil tilled by a 'dirt farmer'. However, the general usage where 'dirt' and 'dirty' are contrasted with 'clean' works in a different kind of way. That will now be our focus.

'Dirty' – like 'damaged', 'chipped' or 'dented' – implies a short-coming of some kind. There is an implicit reference to an ideal, unblemished, normal state and to a deviation from that state.[3] The implication is that dirty objects *require* cleaning. Moreover, typically we are not required to give our grounds for preferring the normal state to the anomaly. In contrast, while it is not impossible that we might *wish* for an item to be dirty or damaged, that would always call for an explanation. Rock musicians sometimes say they want a dirty sound. This must be understood against an acknowledged background where tidiness is the *general* norm.

'Dirty' is also analogous with 'damaged' in another way. The logically primary notion in this usage is not dirt as a *substance* but the underlying object's *quality* of being dirty or soiled. It is a quality that appears when two elements combine: an unwanted substance makes contact with some item perceived as standing in need of protection. The additive collects on the original item, sticks to it or – as with liquids – blends into it. Dirt in this general sense certainly consists of matter, but it is 'dirt' because of its relation to the master object. Analogously, an object is *wet* when water is applied to it and stays on as moisture. Moisture consists of a substance, namely water, but water only becomes moisture by uniting with some other substance (clothes, hair, air and so on).

A substance is dirt only when seen in relation to the soiled object. One consequence of this is that it would involve a contradiction in terms if one tried *in advance* to compose a list of all dirty substances[4] – not even to mention the obviously absurd idea of producing a chemical formula for 'dirt'. In this sense, Justus von Liebig was right in (reportedly) saying, '*Für die Chemie gibt es keinen Dreck*' (for chemistry, no turd exists). The whole science of chemistry is informed by the notion of a *chemical substance*. Chemical substances are analysed in terms of what *they* consist of, taken for themselves and apart from their wider context of use. As soon as a speck of dirt is subjected to analysis it is treated simply as a substance and its dirtiness 'disappears'. Dirt lacks independent identity, which also implies that one cannot purposely produce dirt – in the now relevant sense of the word – and save it in heaps or cardboard boxes for later use.[5] The inherent contradiction in such scenarios was (I take it, consciously) highlighted in the *Dirt Windows* series by artist James Croak, represented at the 'Dirt' exhibition at the

Wellcome Collection, London, in 2011. The artist, according to the catalogue description, 'casts dirt into the form of a window', resulting in black objects the size and shape of a window pane. These *clean* objects of a hard, brick-like quality are the result of collecting 'dirt' and working on 'dirt',[6] but somewhere in the process what once was dirt has turned into recycled, *pure* substance.[7]

In soiling, the additive turns into dirt by sticking to the master object in some way or other. In chemical terms, it must adhere to the adjacent substance or, with liquids, mix with the substance but not completely dissolve into it. The stickier the additive, the more easily it soils object surfaces – which is why Sartre singled out treacle as a particularly Angst-inducing foodstuff.[8] This general principle rules out compact or granular substances as candidates for dirt – such as pieces of wood or grains of sand. For instance, dandruff does not qualify as dirt in this sense. Dusty is not the same as dirty, but dust on a surface may turn into dirt when moistened. Conversely, dirt may dry on a surface, leaving a crust that later dissolves to dust. The requirement of sticking to the object also implies that liquids as such do not constitute *dirt* even though they may be *dirty* and leave dirty stains as well as polluting other liquids. Dishwater counts as dirty more or less by definition, but not as dirt. The other implicit requirement is that, in order to count as dirt, the additive must not be completely absorbed or dissolved into the master object. Air outdoors is usually not called dirty but perhaps polluted or impure (during rush hours in a city); indoors it may count as stuffy or bad. The anomalous state must be thought of as reversible to some extent – through cleaning or, with liquids, through sieving and skimming. If the condition appears permanent we start instead to think of it as inherent in the substance of the master object, now describing the object as *discoloured*, *polluted* or *ruined*.

Master object and additive

These descriptions imply a hierarchical relation between the master object and the additive. The master object is treated as valuable or interesting in its own right while the additive is reduced to its role as a disturbing element.

The characteristic relation between master object and additive is perhaps best understood in terms of the Scholastic, originally Aristotelian, notions of *substance* and *accident*. 'Substance' has since the Middle Ages acquired further meanings that the reader must now ignore: in philosophy (meaning unspecified 'stuff') and in police reports (meaning drugs). The original distinction of substance and accident highlights the difference between qualities that essentially belong to an object and ones somehow added to it. In the present context, the identity, essence or substance of the object is summed up in the description of its 'normal state', which means its rightful, normatively correct state. Accidents like dirt, damage and wear and tear do not alter the essence of the underlying substance.

Thomas Leddy makes use of precisely this contrast between substance and accident in his paper on 'everyday surface aesthetic qualities'.[9] He describes 'dirty' as 'a *surface* quality'. By this he does not just mean that dirt collects on the surfaces of objects. A liquid may be dirty through and through. In the case of greasy hair, one typically cannot point to dirt on a particular surface; it is the hair's general condition that counts. These judgements nevertheless involve the general idea that one should distinguish between the given substance in itself and whatever is added. For Leddy, 'dirty' is a surface quality insofar as it can be kept analytically distinct from the fundamental 'underlying form or substance' of the master object. Considerations of this kind distinguish dirt from a number of other unwanted elements such as trash, refuse, rubbish, garbage and faeces – incidentally, a distinction not honoured in a number of influential accounts of the concepts of dirt and impurity.[10] A 'trashy' object *is* trash or is *like* trash, but a dirty object is not itself dirt. On the contrary, the implication is that the object needs cleaning precisely because it is something *different* from dirt.

Among 'everyday surface aesthetic qualities', Leddy includes *neat, messy, clean* and *dirty*. These qualities require an underlying structure that is tidied up, made a mess of, cleaned or soiled.[11] Correspondingly, the definition of 'tidy' and 'clean' as surface qualities implies that the aesthetically most important function of our tidying and cleaning efforts is to *uncover an underlying form*. 'For example, neatening up or cleaning a facade or a room may reveal an underlying structure with its own aesthetic properties.'[12] The idea that neatness helps us discern the true qualities of things underpinned the aesthetics of white typical of early Functionalist architecture. Against a layer of white enamel paint, according to Functionalist pioneer Le Corbusier, '*everything shows itself as it is*.'[13]

The background assumption in our judgements about soiling must be that the master object is in principle possible to clean, that it in some sense *needs* to be cleaned and is *worth* cleaning.[14] Perhaps this is why bits of toilet paper are typically not described as dirty but as *used*. We do not think there is an underlying substance worth cleaning; of course cleaning is hardly even practically possible in this case. Used toilet paper is called dirty mainly when it may soil *other* objects. The normative position outlined here implies a judgement concerning the relative values of the (valuable) master object and the (worthless) additive. On the other hand, it does not always require a fixed set of priorities. If food falls down it may ruin the carpet, but at other times we say *food* is ruined when it falls on the carpet.

Varieties of badness

This discussion suggests three conclusions which will now be explored further.

1. Dirt can only be conceptualized in its relation to the master object;
2. Dirt-related concepts are defined *teleologically*;
3. The judgement whether an item is clean or dirty is always tied up with a context or situation.

Now to some clarifications:

1. *Dirt(iness) and the master object.* Every master object is dirty or clean in its own ways – just as 'damaged' means different things depending on the kind of thing where damage appears. For each and every object, to know what kind of an object it is is, among other things, to know how it might be soiled, sustain damage or otherwise deviate from its normal state. This understanding also shows in our choice of cleaning methods. Sandpaper may be used for cleaning a piece of wood but not a CD. Freeing a garment, a record player or hair from dirt not only requires that we pay attention to the quality of the offensive substance but that we have some general understanding of the kinds of thing the master objects are.

    The identity of the master object is in turn tied up with ideas of what it is to lead a life in which it has a place. Here it is no doubt important that many of the objects of which we make these judgements are artefacts, purposely made with a function in mind. However, owing to human ingenuity, possible uses for artefacts typically go far beyond the manufacturer's original intentions – consider the use of CDs as scarecrows, the use of clothes pegs by musicians to keep sheet music in place and, in general, the employment of more or less anything as a decorative element in a home.

2. *Teleology.* Concepts and descriptions are teleological if they are internally related to the idea of a goal or telos. This

is not, however, to say we must be able to specify the desirable end state in positive terms. Our implicit understanding of the ideal often shows itself simply in our recognition of shortcomings.

In his *Metaphysics* Aristotle asked what kinds of substance are such that they can imaginably sustain damage. According to him, the description 'damaged' or 'mutilated' is only applicable to substances (objects and living beings) if they are 'wholes' and not merely 'totals'. 'Wholes' are unities consisting of several parts that belong together in a systematic way. For instance, a cup with a handle is a 'whole' but *water* is not – 'the whole water' could only mean something like, 'the whole *cup of* water'. To be mutilated, according to Aristotle, 'things must be such as in virtue of their essence have a certain position'; the essence of the thing determines the internal order of its parts.[15] In plain English this means, for instance: lopping off an arm would be a quick way for a person to lose weight. However, a man with an arm missing has not merely lost a few pounds but falls short of the human essence, man being defined as a biped with two arms. In this respect, living beings and most artefacts are different from materials like water or wax, which allow for increase and diminution without their substance being altered. (Aristotle points out that *numbers* are also incapable of sustaining damage, but this is for the opposite reason: when a number is 'diminished', the number changes entirely.) In sum, the concept of damage involves the idea of a misfit between the current state of the object and its essence.

The teleologically required state of any item is not *one* thing. The same object may enter human activities and practices in various ways and take on many functions (or fail in them). Consequently, our cleaning efforts are not merely dictated by pragmatic considerations. In most cases, cleaning has more to do with aesthetics in a broad sense. For instance, the enjoyment that we derive from a freshly cleaned window is hardly just a matter of the practical usefulness of an unimpeded line of sight through the glass pane. We appreciate the feeling of how the boundary between indoors and outdoors suddenly seems to disappear, the feeling of letting the spring inside the house.

3. *Contextuality.* – 'Are your hands clean?' – I may have to respond to this question by asking what I am expected to *do* with my hands. 'Is X clean?' may take on quite different meanings, and this is because of differences concerning the assumed role of the master object. These things are asked for a reason, not out of a general wish to survey the state of the world.

Consider a somewhat analogous question. A fish is wet when the fisherman draws it into his vessel. But are the fish also wet in their own element, the sea? Perhaps we are inclined to answer 'Yes', but the whole question is distinctly fishy. 'Wet' usually applies to situations where a meaningful contrast can be made between dry and wet things, not to fish in their natural habitat. We will wonder why you would be asking, and before we know *that* we cannot give you a confident answer.

Something similar is true of the question, 'Is X clean or dirty?' The right answer to 'Is that cup clean or dirty?' is 'clean' when I am sitting with a teacup in my lap, waiting for a few drops more, and 'dirty' when you collect it to take to the sink with everyone's cups and saucers.[16] The transformation of my teacup from clean to dirty may look mysterious, for it did not coincide with any visible physical change in the item itself. Should we say there *was* no change after all? Or should we say the transition was merely conventional or symbolic – an idea often favoured in theoretical discussions of dirt and pollution?

What we need to see here is that the change of situational context is just as 'real' as any physical change would be. There is no contradiction involved in saying correctly that 'dirty' and 'clean' are real qualities of objects, *and* saying that what correctly counts as clean in one situation may correctly count as dirty in another. The apparent contradiction would only by created by the implicit assumption that the question, 'Is the cup dirty?' has a completely fixed meaning, staying the same regardless of situation.

This kind of context dependence is often overlooked, here and elsewhere, because the background of the questions we ask in everyday life is for the most part obvious. At the tea party I would *know* whether you are serving more tea or collecting the china. But introduce some ambiguity and the situation changes again. Consider the question of whether a *tree* is dirty. If this is asked out of the blue, and nothing tells us why, the reasonable analysis is that the question has not really been raised yet. For the time being we are not told *why* it is asked, and consequently we do not know what would qualify as a good answer. What is the purpose of a tree? Should it simply grow in the forest? Is it a decorative element in the garden, future timber and firewood or a place for climbing? But real communication is never characterized by such radical openness of interpretation. Suppose a child wants to climb a wet tree in his Sunday best. Is the tree dirty? The question would present no difficulties at all, and we would not be tempted to think it is all just subjective. What we have here is interplay between object and situation: the situation determines what is expected of the object, while the identity of the object determines what kinds of situation it *may* be involved in.

Primary and secondary master objects

The master object may also be judged from the point of view of the teleology of some *other* object. Often what motivates the judgement is not concern for the state of the object as such, but the worry that the dirty object may soil something else. The question 'Are your hands clean?' is almost invariably asked with such concerns in mind. This of course has to do with the unique role of human hands in the handling or manipulation of objects. My assessment of whether, for instance, moisturizer would make my hands dirty is dependent on what I am planning to do next: what kinds of soiling would be unacceptable on the things I will be touching.

It is helpful to have this distinction fixed by introducing terms for *primary* and *secondary* master objects. Dirt appears when an additive attaches to a master object, disturbing or clouding its essence, ideal state or *telos*. Now we should add: in soiling, either the *telos* of the object (now the *primary* master object) is disturbed by the unwanted additive; *or* there is a risk that the affected object (now the *secondary* master object) might interfere with the *telos* of something else (a primary master object). The *telos* of the *primary* master object is, in both cases, what ultimately defines the situation as one of soiling. While primary master objects are cleaned and protected against dirt for their own sake, secondary master objects are cleaned when they would otherwise risk soiling a primary master object.

For illustration, consider what happens when my shoes are ruined on a muddy forest walk. The ground counts as dirty because my shoes are to be protected. But when I reach home my shoes now count as the dirty item while the carpet becomes the element that needs protection. This demonstrates that the distinction between primary and secondary master objects is not one between *objects* of different kinds, but between two kinds of role that an object may take on as a carrier of dirt. At the same time, certain objects more typically appear in the one role than in the other. Human faces and, for instance, spectacles typically appear as primary master objects and much more seldom as secondary. They are usually cleaned for their own sake. In contrast, substances like vomit are difficult even to imagine as primary master objects of dirt. With the possible exception of research in medicine and healthcare, we have no conception of a difference between a first-class and a deficient sample, nor do we quite know what would be required for cleaning *it*, as opposed to cleaning it *up* from a floor.

Degrees of soiling

The fact that each object has its own ways of being clean and dirty creates difficulties for any quantitative comparison. Mostly we would just compare the condition of the same object before and after cleaning or, as with two white shirts, the conditions of distinct but qualitatively similar objects. If the two items are completely different in kind, the idea of comparing their degrees of soiling would invite the question of why a comparison should be relevant in the first place. The reason may come in the form of a connecting link, for instance when you say, 'The water is even worse than the shirt.' It is no use washing the shirt *there*, perhaps because it has already been used for washing too many other garments.

For the sake of argument, try to imagine a universal, quantitative scale from absolutely dirty to absolutely clean, with a slot in readiness for each and every object imaginable. Earth, streets and floors would be placed somewhere close to the lower end and sterilized surgical instruments towards the upper end. Any attempt to construe such a scale would, however, be thoroughly misleading. The state that counts as dirty for one object might be the normal, unblemished state for another. A meticulously cleaned floor would probably carry more alien particles than an unwashed surgical knife. Usually 'a clean floor' is simply a floor that a guest would find aesthetically pleasing – the requirement is not that it should be safely placed in contact with open wounds. In fact, a medically speaking healthy floor arguably *ought* to carry a certain quantity of dust and microbes in order to prevent the development of allergies in children. Even for the same object, judgements would have to differ depending on the context.

The idea of a quantitative scale of cleanliness involves a further complication. If it were carried to its logical conclusion, *no* element except absolute vacuum would ever count as completely clean; only pure nothingness would do. André Comte-Sponville states exactly this in his work *A Small Treatise on the Great Virtues*:

> What is pure is clean, spotless, unsoiled. Pure water is unmixed water, water that is nothing but water. Note that such water is actually dead, a fact that says a lot about life and about a certain nostalgia for purity. Whatever lives also soils, and all that cleans kills. Thus we add chlorine to our swimming pools. Purity is impossible; we can only choose between different varieties of impurities, and the practice of this choice we call hygiene ... Purity ... is on the side of death and nothingness. Water is pure when it contains no germs, chlorine, calcium, or mineral salts and is nothing but water – in other words, a water that does not exist, or rather that exists only in laboratories. Such water, odorless and tasteless, would kill us if we drank nothing else. Furthermore, it is pure on only one level. If the hydrogen molecules could speak, they could protest their contamination by oxygen, and each nucleus could complain of being forced into an impure association with an electron. Only nothingness is pure, and nothingness is nothing: whatever exists is a stain on the infinite void, and all existence is impure.[17]

I would not agree with the author of *A Small Treatise* (of 368 pages). Freedom from dirt is not the same as hygiene or homogeneity, conditions to which his description is in part applicable.

Chlorinated water is clean in the sink. Sea water, with salt and microscopic life, is clean in the sea. For Comte-Sponville both of these *clean* cases would count as impure or unclean water. He has apparently been led astray by misleading analogies with the concept of chemical purity or homogeneity. The chemical purity of a substance may be expressed quantitatively; in that context, absolute purity would imply the total absence of foreign substance. The conclusion 'purity does not exist'[18] follows from the identification of purity with absolute purity, not so much an existing or attainable state as an ideal limit for chemical analysis.

The relation between chemical purity and purity as cleanness is more properly seen as analogous with the relation between the concept of geometrical size and the concepts of 'big' and 'small'. 'Big' and 'small' are undoubtedly *related to* practices of geometrical measurement, but unlike geometry they do not allow for the construction of a universal scale. If you lose a *big* pencil inside a *small* car, no paradox is involved. Applying Wittgenstein's phrase, two different language games are being played.

Clean and dirty, pure and impure

'Dirty' is contrasted with 'clean' but also with 'pure'. 'Pure', in turn, sometimes contrasts with 'dirty' and 'polluted' and sometimes with 'mixed'. When water is 'pure' it is either *free of dirt* or *unmixed*. Tap water is free of dirt but it may contain additives. Water in an undisturbed mountain lake is free of additives but not necessarily of dirt, while distilled water is free of both.

A lump of *pure* gold – unmixed, unadulterated gold – may be *dirty* without any sense of paradox, which indicates that 'dirty' is not synonymous with 'mixed'. This is also true in metaphorical usage. Racially or ethnically pure blood is contrasted with the mixed ancestry of the racially *impure*, not with the racially *dirty*.[19] 'Purity' is in these cases understood as homogeneity. We are familiar with 'pure' in the sense of 'homogeneous', for instance, from expressions like 'pure alcohol', 'a pure sample' and 'pure nonsense' – that is, sheer nonsense, *nothing but* nonsense. A 'pure doctrine' is the unmixed, original, impeccable doctrine.

'Pure' may also stand for an undisturbed, virginal, ideal or original state, as when undisturbed nature is described as pure. The state of primeval purity may, however, be upset by elements coming from the outside. Once the *untouched* state is disturbed it is lost for ever, and its restoration is humanly impossible. Paradise was pure, not clean.[20] 'Clean', in contrast, typically seems to indicate a state *brought about by someone* through cleaning. It is not a primeval state but the result of conscious cleaning efforts. Thus the *activity* of cleaning is the starting point of the logic of cleanliness; a new clean shirt is for the most part a shirt that *has been* washed. What appeals to us in a clean shirt are not only its original qualities but the cleaning operation that lets those qualities shine forth. Leddy remarks at this juncture:

> It is true that when a Monet painting is cleaned we are better able to appreciate the underlying structure and the brilliance of the colours. However, it is often the case that when something is cleaned, we simply appreciate the cleanness of it, particularly if *we* have just cleaned it. There can be considerable pleasure in contemplating something cleaned with great effort. What is appreciated is not simply the object cleaned but that plus a combination of process and product: the cleaning up and the nature of the object cleaned.[21]

It is perhaps possible to say, in a somewhat speculative vein, that the dirty is situated at a point in time between the two unsullied extremes: it lies between the undisturbed and the cleaned. To be cleaned is for the object to return to something *reminiscent of* its original state, but now with the difference that the state is a result of human effort. 'Purification' is also a possible activity, but it seems typically to indicate something more radical than mere cleaning – it is more like making a complete new start.

Depending on context, 'pure' can carry positive, negative and neutral associations. We speak of pure gold, pure nonsense and pure coincidence. However, there are good reasons to think of the positive evaluation as primary and the negative or neutral usages as derived. Phrases like 'pure nonsense' and 'pure coincidence' look like idiomatic expressions where the word 'pure' no longer plays an independent role.[22] Thus while it is possible to say 'this gold is pure' we do not normally say 'this nonsense is pure' or 'this coincidence is pure'. As A.D.M. Walker points out in a paper on this topic, expressions of the type 'this X is pure' seem to presuppose some form of *benevolent interest in the purity of X*.[23] Most of us have no trouble understanding why 'this X is pure' is used for *gold* because we think of gold almost as synonymous with the valuable. We may certainly imagine *some* circumstance where it would also make sense to speak of the purity of mud or of vomit, but only if we have some idea of why such a state should be thought of as worth striving for. On the other hand, benevolent interest in the purity of X does not seem to require that the additive must be seen in a *negative* light. Consider copper mixed with a percentage of gold. Gold is now described as impurity, but this is simply because gold is something *else* other than the material whose purity is being judged.[24]

In the contrast between *pure* and *impure*, sometimes the one and sometimes the other opposite is the primary notion. Sometimes the pure is defined first while the impure is whatever deviates from the pure. For 'pure gold' and 'pure blue', *pure X* is the starting point – unmixed gold and unmixed blue. In this usage, 'pure water' means 'H_2O and nothing else', while 'impure water' is 'H_2O plus an admixture'. Sometimes the logic for ascriptions of purity works the other way around. The speaker has some *specific* impurity in mind and 'purity' is defined as absence of the noxious substance. Benevolent interest in the purity of X must be assumed, but now the procedure for judging is different: it starts with an assessment of what kinds of additive to X are *disturbing*. A.D.M. Walker considers the example of 'air in North Wales'. To say that the air is pure in North Wales is not to say it is air and nothing but air but rather that it does not carry disturbing or damaging substances.[25] 'Pure water' in this second kind of sense is water free of pollution. Similarly, Walker points out that when a vessel is impure, the implication is not that it partly *consists of* something else than a vessel; rather the vessel holds something that should not be there.

Someone's behaviour may be described as pure game or a mere game, where the implication is that, contrary to appearances, it is nothing but a game and should not be taken at face value. On the other hand, when an actual game of football is 'pure', the point is not that the game is game and nothing else. Rather, it is free of disturbing elements such as cheating – the opposite being an impure or, worse still, a dirty game.

Dirt and relativity

The fact that different individuals and cultures are not in agreement in their reactions to dirt is often, in theoretical debate, used to motivate the conclusion that dirt is relative – 'it exists in the eye of the beholder'.[26] However, the previous analysis suggests that disagreements about soiling are frequently connected with ambiguities about context – about the identity of the object and its role in the situation at hand. In order to understand in what sense dirt is 'relative' it is consequently a good idea to distinguish between two forms of disagreement:

1. Disagreements based on differences of *sensitivity* to dirt;
2. Disagreements based on different ways of judging the *object* in question; which may be further divided as follows:
a. Differences with regard to the identification of the object as such;

b. Differences with regard to the role of the object in the specific situation;

c. Differences about *which* specific aspect of the object's role in the situation should be relevant.

With regard to sensitivity to dirt, I am inclined to think our differences are smaller than commonly assumed. In any case, variations of tolerance do not imply disagreement about facts. Quite the contrary: if we speak of differences of sensitivity or tolerance we are already presuming *constant* qualities of things, qualities to which people react differently. Precisely because our sensitivities differ, 'dirty' cannot simply be identified with whatever crosses the threshold of tolerance for a particular individual or culture. Dirt nevertheless remains relative in another sense: it is relative to variable conceptions of the master object.

Our methods of determining whether a thing is clean or dirty indicate *what* kind of a thing we take it to be. Thus the question of whether a refrigerator needs cleaning is usually settled by looking inside and not by checking the condition of the back side, which for the most part (apart from very heavy collections of dust) is not immediately relevant to its functioning. On the other hand, the identity of the master object frequently allows for ambiguities which may even be consciously exploited. The classical example is the non-commissioned officer who chastises newly enlisted soldiers for not dusting the top side of the barrack room door.

Another, culturally more interesting, case has been related by Anna Magdalena Midtgaard, working at the Rare Books section of Copenhagen Royal Library.[27] Ideas of what constitutes dirt on a given object reflect our ideas about what *naturally belongs* to it and what counts as an alien addition. Midtgaard brings this out in a paper on the conservation of books. Major libraries today have custom-made vacuum cleaners for books, and there are also techniques for washing and ironing book pages. Some librarians find it important as far as possible to remove stains and dust from old volumes, thinking of the *new* volume as the ideal. Others would take a more conservational approach. Grains of pollen and sand may be seen as belonging to the volume's history. They sometimes contain useful information about its place of origin and the hands through which it has reached its present location. The variety of existing attitudes among librarians reflects not only differences of taste, toleration and sensibilities, but ideas about the identity of the item itself. A stain may either be seen as a blemish or as patina: either as external to the volume or as a natural feature of it. Technically speaking, patina is indistinguishable from wear and dirt, but describing it as 'patina' implies that it would be barbaric to remove it. The old manuscript volume must be able to give us the message 'I am five hundred years old'; but it need not necessarily cry out 'I was *new* five hundred years ago.'

Ambiguities about the nature of a master object sometimes trace the distinction between *indoors* and *outdoors*, which shows variation across cultures. Different perceptions of this distinction might sometimes explain hygienic horror stories told by tourists. Consider the reports by returning visitors to Eternal Russia about its eternally filthy, eternally nicotine-marinated staircases – reports often wrongly putting the problem down to Socialist heritage, despite the fact that the situation was the same under the Tsars and has hardly improved since the end of the Cold War. It would be equally unfair to accuse some atavistic quality of the Broad Slavic Soul, especially considering the stark contrast between the untidy staircase and the spotless and cosy inside of the flats themselves. One does wonder why a country that has the technology to send its citizens to outer space (and often back again) has not got its act together on what might look like a minor hygienic challenge.

The explanation might be sought in the conceptualization of living space. In northwest Europe the staircase is apparently understood as a continuation of the actual flat towards the outside of the building, while Russians seem to operate with the idea of the stairs as an extended street, ending only at the apartment door. This is a conceptual distinction that now, with the privatization of previously municipally owned apartments, has also in effect been written down as law. While the flats themselves are private, the facade and the staircase still belong to the municipality.[28] This is a nice illustration of a general point: our concepts and our social relations are merely two sides of a coin.[29] Instances of different conceptualizations of living space can also be seen, perhaps less dramatically, within Western Europe: there are different ideas about where to lay carpets, where smoking is normal and whether to take off one's shoes indoors.

Different teleologies may also work at cross purposes within one and the same culture. A factory pollutes nature when it leaks chlorine – otherwise used as *detergent* – into a river. Conversely, the very same industrial establishment must be defended against natural dirt. Thus it needs protection from the untouched nature that needs protection against *it*.

Living beings, lifeless things, everyday objects

In moral philosophy, living beings are sometimes described as entities that 'have a *welfare*'. Living beings have needs that call for attention; they can be treated ill or well. 'Guinness is good for you,' if indeed it is, because you are a being of the kind of which it can be said that things can be good or bad for, or go well or badly for. The fact that living beings have a welfare is perhaps best seen when they suffer. We can, for instance, immediately tell when a potted plant has been neglected. The plant must be watered, not because someone wants it that way but because, as a living thing, the plant has a welfare.

It appears that also many 'lifeless' ordinary objects have a welfare. Things can go well or badly for them, and they require attention from us. Someone might call this an anthropomorphic or 'biomorphic' suggestion, ascribing to things qualities that only belong to living beings. Before going any further I must respond to this, and the response consists of two points.

First of all, 'having a welfare' is not really a *quality*. It is not possible to establish the presence of any such extraordinary quality through some sort of completely neutral observation of reality. In this context, welfare is rather a perspective, an aspect under which a number of phenomena are viewed. The proof of the perspective lies in its possibilities of use. To ask whether an entity 'has' a welfare is consequently to ask whether it is *meaningful* to understand it from the perspective of welfare; whether anything is gained or lost in the process. Secondly, calling a perspective of this kind anthropomorphic or biomorphic would amount to the implicit suggestion that *only* human beings or living beings are entities properly to be seen as subjects of welfare. But *that* has, of course, not been established – on the contrary, I have already pointed to numerous obviously *meaningful* ways of describing 'lifeless' objects within the framework of that kind of teleology.

Thus it is plausible to say that human thinking, in addition to the categories of living beings and 'mere' objects, also counts on a third category: that of objects with a *telos* or purpose. This creates the framework for a language in which objects can be described as damaged and mended, dishevelled and tidy, dirty and clean. We normally know, of a particular artefact, that it has been produced with an eye on certain possibilities of use, so that its uses appear to be more or less built into the item itself as potentialities. For instance, a factory that makes knives and forks is not merely producing 'physical objects' for consumers to subsequently identify and figure out uses for. These items are produced in the first place only because their identity is settled from the start. As soon as we describe the item at hand as a *fork* we have already rooted it in a discourse of practical possibilities, a discourse that would of course look different if we were instead merely to refer to it as 'an object with pointed ends' or 'an object made of aluminium'.[30] It is, in most cases, quite natural and easy for us to identify what it would be proper to expect of a fork – for instance, how to recognize dirt and damage on it. There is a relationship between things and us, a mutual agreement that neither of us is supposed to break.

Judgements about soiling are, in one sense, *value* judgements; above all in the sense that, in the normal case and by definition, clean is better than dirty. In another sense they are judgements of facts. Whether we should stress the one or the other aspect – *that* question is, I take it, a matter of the specific issue that we want to address. In a somewhat similar way, 'I owe you £10' may be treated both as a factual description and as a normative statement.[31] The bottom line is that our general ability to identify objects as 'clean' or 'dirty' is an aspect of our ability to identify objects in the first place. The identity of a given object is determined by its essence, point or *telos*.

It is easy to see that this analysis can be generalized beyond just the question of soiling. Our general perception of the material environment contains an Aristotelian element, that of a distinction between substance and accident. And it also (without contradicting the previous point) contains an element of Platonism. Our experience of the world is shaped by ideas of perfection and of falling short of perfection. It is internally structured by a notion of value or of the Good – not in opposition to facts but itself a condition of the meaningful perception of facts.[32]

FOUR

Reductionism and the Role of Science

How are ordinary objects possible?

The Monist – a well-known journal of professional philosophy – published an issue in 2005 on 'ordinary objects'. This is an example of its editorial policy of devoting entire issues to themes currently under intense debate. In its title, one of the contributed essays sums up the crucial question: 'How are Ordinary Objects Possible?'[1] Discussion continues as I am writing. By 'ordinary objects' we should understand things like tables, screwdrivers, lutes, chestnuts and horses. Sometimes the chosen example appears to be just whatever the writer happened to clap his or her eyes on at the time of writing. This is understandable because nothing very much hangs on precisely *which* ordinary objects are chosen for treatment at this very general level.

Non-philosophers might wonder how on earth the existence of ordinary objects should be regarded as a problem in the first place. I have some sympathy with this. For one thing, it seems fair to say that the very concept of 'object' is in itself largely framed on the model of ordinary objects. Hence one should think that ordinary objects would be among the last entities whose existence would be called into question. On the other hand, the relevance of a philosophical problem is always a function of the general state of philosophy, including philosophical thinking on areas generally *not* treated as philosophically problematic. Thus we should not try to decide in the abstract whether the existence of ordinary objects should be called a *real* problem or a 'pseudo-problem', but rather we need to see under what conditions it would show up a problematic aspect. A problem is real as long as the intellectual conditions are there which contribute to its being a problem.

The background question, especially given the present state of scientific knowledge, is whether we can still justifiably think of the world as being made up of stable ordinary objects. In the last analysis, will the belief in medium-sized dry goods turn out to be misleading in the same way as the belief in sunrises once did?[2] Astronomically, the sun does not rise – the spot of the earth's surface where the observer stands simply turns eastwards to face the sun – but we may keep the word 'sunrise' as a harmless turn of phrase. Are ordinary objects too something like that – harmless fictions? (But can we even imagine what *that* would mean?) The emergence of a problem of ordinary objects is connected with the current state of mainstream metaphysics, which has consciously aligned itself with (natural) science and the kind of world view assumed to be inherent in it. And it must be conceded that 'ordinary object' is not a *scientific* concept. If science is the starting point for ontology, why should we assume anything to exist in time and space except atoms?[3]

In his contribution to the journal volume, John Heil quotes the now famous, or infamous, description of this conundrum included in the physicist A. S. Eddington's book *The Nature of the Physical World* (1928). When Eddington starts writing he moves, he tells us, his two chairs next to his two tables and then takes up his two pens. This is because there are 'duplicates' of each of these familiar items. His one table is an old acquaintance since many years, 'a commonplace object of that environment which I call the world'. The other is more problematic:

> Table No. 2 is my scientific table . . . My scientific table is mostly emptiness. Sparsely scattered in that emptiness are numerous electric charges rushing about with great speed; but their combined bulk amounts to less than a billionth

of the bulk of the table itself. Notwithstanding its strange construction it turns out to be an entirely efficient table. It supports my writing paper as satisfactorily as table No. 1; for when I lay the paper on it the little electric particles with their headlong speed keep on hitting the underside, so that the paper is maintained in shuttlecock fashion at a nearly steady level.[4]

But further, 'modern physics has by delicate test and remorseless logic assured me that my second scientific table is the only one which is really there'.[5] In his essay, Heil uses Eddington as a starting point and asks whether tables really exist. His final answer is a cautious Yes, but Heil frames his question in the following way:

> When we looked closely at the table, we observed a swarm . . . Our best science tells us that the swarm exists, behaves in particular ways, and falls under strict laws of nature. The table's standing is less impressive. Physics includes no mention of tables. Whenever we look closely at a table, it seems to dissolve, turning into a swarm.[6]

Meteorology tells us that clouds are swarms of tiny drops of water. Supposedly in the same way, the table is identified as a swarm of tiny particles. In both cases, the crucial operation that shows us the truth is described as an act of *moving closer*. However, Heil's use of this metaphor is quite obviously misleading. Taken literally, the description would be right concerning the cloud but wrong concerning the table. It would actually be impossible to discover that a table is a swarm by 'looking closely' – although we might find out other facts about what it is made of; perhaps chipboard instead of solid wood. Using magnifying devices like an electron microscope might in an attenuated sense qualify as 'looking closely' – even though our eyes are not literally brought closer to the object. What we see in an electron microscope is a moot point, for the apparatus actually produces the image we see rather than simply magnifying an existing view. In any case, the electron microscope was developed *after*, and as one application of, the conception of matter as consisting of elementary particles.

This might look like a pedantic observation from my part, but it highlights the profound difference between the cloud of water drops and the swarm of elementary particles. That a particular cloud consists of water drops is a straightforward empirical discovery. The statement that a table, like everything else, consists of elementary particles is more like a *requirement* we make because of the general role that the concept of particle has in physics. This is not to say that it is empirically unfounded, but it does mean that a systematic theoretical background is assumed. It could not, for instance, be merely a discovery about tables as opposed to other furniture; nor could it be a discovery about just this one table. The idea at play here is not merely an application of the everyday practical notion of a thing 'consisting of' something or other. A table consists *either* of wood *or* of concrete *or* of some other material, but elementary particles would not figure as *materials* in this list of alternatives. In order to make a cloud I can use water vapour; in order to make a table I can use wood, concrete and so on; and I can use elementary particles in order to make, well, what?

Even the reasons for investigating clouds and investigating tables would be different. The discovery that clouds consist of tiny drops was the scientific response to previous ignorance about what clouds are. The statement that tables consist of particles is not a response to ignorance about what tables are. On the other hand, there are other legitimate questions about what kind of a thing a table is or what kind of a material wood is; and the best metaphor in some cases might not be that of looking more closely but of creating *distance*, for instance, in the form of an *overview* – of, say, the ecosystem of a forest.[7]

Like most philosophers contributing to this particular debate, Heil certainly concludes that we are at least in some qualified sense *justified* in assuming the real existence of ordinary objects. One might think this is good news, but of course it still betrays the author's basic worry that ordinary objects need defending – that they are in some sense outlaws until there is an account of them in terms of scientific metaphysics. The philosopher Lynne Rudder Baker suggests, for instance, that a scientifically acceptable metaphysics of ordinary objects is needed as a rational underpinning of legal property rights.[8] From my point of view, the debate shows that the very idea of an ordinary object must become dubious if philosophy looks to science for ideological guidance.

Dirt: two kinds of reductionism

The existence of ordinary objects being granted, there is still the question of *how* they exist. Problems start when things in our environment are conceptualized *primarily* or *at bottom* as physical or material objects, like collections of matter, as opposed to everyday objects like tables and clothing. The idea behind that kind of conceptualization would be that objects are only later endowed with distinct functions and purposes; through subjective operations that do not touch their *real* identities. If objects at bottom are meaningless and functionless, in what kinds of circumstance can it be meaningful to ascribe purposes to objects (for instance, to a table or to garments) or to non-independent parts of living creatures (to human hands, to animal fur)?

If we want *inherent* purposes, natural science appears to answer quite simply: 'under *no* circumstances'. In science, objects have purposes only to the extent that they are *given* such through the action of human (and perhaps other animate) beings. During the last three or four centuries, science has been shedding its Aristotelian past. In the process it has been steadily and methodically purging itself of explanations in terms of purpose, replacing them wherever possible with causal or functional explanations. While the project has not been equally successful across the board, its agenda has at least been stated in every science. For many, extending the range of causal explanations and getting rid of teleology is the key to theoretical advancement in all research. Nature has no goals; the appearance of teleology is the result of a limited human perspective, and intellectual progress consists in overcoming such limits.

From a practical point of view, however, this might be a surprising line to take. The descriptions 'clean' and 'dirty' presuppose teleology. Can it really be true that science has no use for them? No one insists more on hygiene than the chemist in the laboratory and the surgeon in the operating theatre. Thus it seems that at least in practice, if not in theory, dirt and soiling *exist* even for the scientist. The requirement of cleanliness is already implicit in the requirements of chemical analysis. Quite simply, *pure* samples are assumed. This is true also in chemical industry, where production according to plan requires pure raw materials. 'Impurity' is here to be defined as any substance that does not properly belong to the production process, while 'pure' substances have exactly the composition that the planned process would require.[9]

These examples indicate at least that teleological thinking of some kind is solidly anchored in applied science, but in a certain sense such responses would still miss the theoretical question. Chemists and engineers speak of purposes and goals because *they* work for purposes and goals, but the examples do not show us *things themselves* having goals. But if it is indeed true that 'dirty' and 'clean' cannot be scientifically validated as real qualities of things we nevertheless face the question of why in practice it *looks as if* judgements about soiling were both meaningful and (often) true.

Consider why we believe cleanliness to be important, and why we engage in specific cleaning operations – immersing objects in water, brushing and scrubbing, keeping clean and dirty objects separate. The most immediate explanation might simply be: my white shirt needs to be washed because the collar is not clean. This would be a valid piece of information if you were just asking me why *this particular* piece of clothing needs washing, but it would not explain why clean shirts are *generally* preferred. Sometimes there is a special reason why I want a clean crisp shirt, for instance because I hope to make a good impression at a job interview. But this of course gives rise to almost the same question once again: why do *interviewers* prefer candidates with clean shirts? Why are clean shirts generally taken to be preferable to soiled ones? Here I feel the impulse to cut the conversation short and say: clean shirts just are superior, full stop. But that would invite the renewed question of what kinds of *way* clean shirts are superior. If I tell you they smell less under the armpits, and so on, the next question would be why *that* should be considered a good thing. In the end, these questions would concern the very point of the language game of 'clean and dirty'.

What this comes down to is the requirement that I should explain the superiority of clean over dirty in some terms *other than* mere general preference for cleanliness. This is in harmony with what 'giving an explanation' generally means: an explanation should point to something else other than the exact thing one is supposed to explain. If I take the demand for an explanation seriously I will have to start on the assumption that, insofar as clean shirts are in fact preferable to dirty ones, it must be either because they have some additional quality still to be described, or because they are useful as a means of achieving some other desirable end.

What is the 'other desirable end'? Two main explanations have been offered; the two explanations may coexist, even reinforce each other on the lines of a mutual benefit society. Both are kinds of reductionism about dirt. On the one hand, there is *hygienic* reductionism: explaining the ideas of soiling and cleanliness in terms of purely medical considerations, thus in terms of human *biology*. On the other hand, *anthropological* reductionism reduces cleanliness to pollution taboos – thus to human *culture*.

Hygienic reductionism

At the first blush it looks as if hygienic reductionism is capable of making at least some part of soiling safe for science. Many hygienic reductionists would say soiling really exists in *some* form, namely, in the form of substances identified as potential carriers of disease. It is only that our ordinary judgements about soiling still belong to a pre-scientific stage of 'folk' theorizing.

Scientific ideas of hygiene were formulated during the last couple of centuries thanks to discoveries by medical men like Louis Pasteur, Ignaz Semmelweis and Joseph Lister – researchers who, around the middle of the nineteenth century, laid the foundations of our modern understanding of contagion. Hygiene as sanitary science strictly speaking comprises more than just aseptic and antiseptic cleanliness, but hygienic cleanliness now belongs to our main methods of combating epidemic diseases. This quite naturally leads us to the question of whether our general hostility to dirt might not also be explained and justified by health concerns.

The assimilation of cleanliness to hygiene is, however, less than compelling as soon as we leave the hospital milieu. I am certainly not washing my white shirt because I fear infection. On this theme I have consulted a brochure by the National Swedish Board of Health and Welfare. The reader is told that we can be relatively unwashed without any hazard to the skin: 'In medical respect, the removal of dirt is in most cases not of any consequence.' On the whole, 'standards of cleanliness in the home are above all a question of what we are personally comfortable with.'[10] The claim is not that washing serves no health purpose at all, for in many situations it is an extremely efficient way to fight contagion. However, cleanliness has obvious additional functions that fall outside hygiene, having more to do with aesthetic and social considerations.

In his work *The Civilizing Process* (1939), Norbert Elias gives us a detailed argument on why cleanliness must be distinguished from hygiene. He argues that, in many cases, considerations we would justify today in the name of hygiene were originally rather a question of what was 'done' or 'not done' in polite society. Spitting was, for instance, condemned as 'indelicate and disgusting' long before there was any understanding of associated health risks.[11]

> It is well to establish once and for all that something which we know to be harmful to health by no means necessarily arouses feelings of distaste or shame. And conversely, something that arouses these feelings need not be at all detrimental to health. Someone who eats noisily or with his hands nowadays arouses feelings of extreme distaste without there being the slightest fear for his health. But neither the thought of someone reading by bad light nor the idea of poison gas, for example, arouses remotely similar feelings of distaste or shame, although the harmful consequences for health are obvious.[12]

We exchange kisses and shake hands. We use public transportation and we even keep cats and dogs in the house despite the documented risks of contagion. On top of this, our aversion to dirt sometimes prompts us to adopt aesthetic solutions that go diametrically against aseptic hygiene. We frequently prefer dark or patterned fabrics and wallpapers precisely because they make soiling less visible on clothes and interior decoration, which is of course also why unmixed white would be the superior colour from a purely hygienic point of view.

Indeed it seems that by 'dirt' we mostly mean visible or otherwise readily discernible soiling. With regard to hygiene, we are instead familiar with the fact that the germs carrying contagion are not obvious to the naked eye. This was a point often made in the early hygienic campaigns of the late nineteenth century: people should above all learn to protect themselves against *invisible* risks lurking in the everyday environment. Some ideas of health hazards in the household are based on the further assumption that dirt and dust, consisting of matter of uncontrollable and often animal origin, can be *supposed* to contain invisible bacteria, virus and mites.

Admittedly, some of our reactions to soiling are related to hygiene. Our instinctive rejection of excrement and spoiled food is quite clearly connected with natural protective reactions against sources of infection.[13] It also makes sense to assume that such reactions were essential to the survival of early hominids. But all of this would fall far short of the claim that our *present* ideas of dirty and clean are mainly motivated by considerations of health hazards. Seeing that the ideas of hygiene and cleanliness pull in two different, sometimes diametrically opposed directions, they must mean different things.

Reforming our ideas of pollution

A possible conclusion might be: our present cleanliness practices are devoid of rational motivation, hence *irrational*. Martha Nussbaum argues that disgust, when not caused by hygienic concerns, depends on symbolic associations rather than rational motives. 'The basic idea', she notes, 'is that past contact between an innocuous substance and a disgust substance causes rejection of the acceptable substance.' This, we are told, is simply 'sympathetic magic', involving a sense of 'psychological contamination'. According to the magical principle, 'things that have been in contact continue ever afterwards to act on one another.'[14]

Would it then perhaps be possible in the future to replace our present, conventional-cum-magical ideas of cleanliness with a scientifically motivated way of life based on real information about things good and bad for the health? Nussbaum argues that 'the moral progress of society can be measured by the degree to which it separates disgust from danger and indignation, basing laws and social rules on *substantive harm*, rather than on the *symbolic relationship* an object bears to anxieties about animality and mortality.'[15] Her overall position on dirt and disgust can be summed up as follows. What *currently* elicits human disgust is largely determined by symbolic associations; but this is a kind of distortion, for the proper objects of disgust are merely the substances likely to be harmful to us. And it is a task for educators and reformers to make people see this. Thus Nussbaum is indicating that we can and, moreover, *ought to* organize our lives more along the lines of scientific hygiene.

Many efforts of the early activists for the welfare state can indeed be traced back to the ideal of implementing scientific hygiene in everyday life. In *Brave New World* (1932), Aldous Huxley gives us a glimpse both of the social conditions that the advocates of social reform encountered and of his own highly critical caricature of their views:

> Home, home – a few small rooms, stiflingly over-inhabited by a man, by a periodically teeming woman, by a rabble of boys and girls of all ages. No air, no space; an understerilized prison; darkness, disease, and smells ... And home was as squalid psychically as physically. Psychically, it was a rabbit hole, a midden, hot with the frictions of tightly packed life, reeking with emotion. What suffocating intimacies, what dangerous, insane, obscene relationships between the members of the family group! Maniacally, the mother brooded over her children (*her* children) ... brooded over them like a cat over its kittens; but a cat that could talk, a cat that could say, 'My baby, my baby,' over and over again. 'My baby, and oh, oh, at my breast, the little hands, the hunger, and that unspeakable agonizing pleasure! Till at last my baby sleeps, my baby sleeps with a bubble of white milk at the corner of his mouth. My little baby sleeps ...' 'Yes,' ... 'you may well shudder.'[16]

As in many utopian and dystopian novels of the time, in *Brave New World* human dwellings are standardized. Huxley was connecting his forecast of future reforms with the intense contemporary debate on working-class living conditions and the sanitization of entire urban neighbourhoods. The battle cry was: 'Light and Air to Everyone!' This would go hand in hand with spreading hygienic awareness among the general public. It would be unfair to associate Nussbaum directly with the compulsive hygiene in evidence in *Brave New World*; on the whole she advocates higher tolerance of dirt. But she certainly shares the belief in social engineering and like early twentieth-century reformers she defends the general idea of a rational, scientifically informed revision of our attitudes to soiling.

Could human societies ever be completely reshaped according to the prescriptions of medical hygiene? Regardless of whether we would find such reforms desirable or even possible, the fact remains that hygiene and cleanliness are essentially distinct. It appears possible to define hygiene in completely functional terms. The neglect of hygiene in hospitals, industrial kitchens or laboratories would put their very functioning at risk. But apart from those restricted milieus of rather recent origin, life *without* medical hygiene is not only imaginable but for the most part quite similar to the lives we are already living. Life without the concepts of dirt and cleanliness is, however, a different matter. To imagine *that* would be to imagine our lives as completely overturned. Paradoxically, we cannot do without cleanliness precisely because cleanliness, unlike medical hygiene, is not a response to any *specific* need. It is a goal in itself.

Anthropological reductionism

The shortcomings of hygienic reductionism may be invoked as an argument for an opposite form of reductionism. If our normal cleaning activities are not always demonstrably good for the physical health, perhaps they are good for some other, less tangible purpose? Could it be that our relationship to soiling is merely a symbolic representation of something quite different? Anthropological reductionism is the currently most favoured approach to dirt and impurity.

For anthropological reductionism about dirt, dirt in the every-day sense does not really exist in the world. The question of what kinds of qualities *really* exist is something that anthropological reductionism prefers to pass on to science. But the fact remains that *we*, human beings, *consider* certain things to be dirty or clean. The focus now moves on from facts about the world to the human being who, either instinctively or as a learned response, projects her hopes and fears upon an originally neutral, physical reality.

Anthropological reductionism elaborates the main idea that the meaning of the word 'dirty' is more closely related to socially defined status, such as 'forbidden', than to physical descriptive expressions like 'rusty', 'discoloured' or 'damaged'. One prominent example is found in Sigmund Freud's discussion of the concept of purity and the associated idea of projection. In this connection, it is good to keep in mind that Freud personally thought of himself first and foremost as a natural scientist. As a medical doctor, he did not believe that our rejection of dirt in everyday life had any good hygienic explanation. Actions that people wished to justify in the name of hygiene were frequently expressions of fears and concerns whose roots grew elsewhere in a much darker kind of soil. Consider Freud's attempt, in *Totem and Taboo* (first published in 1913), to account for our perception of 'the uncanny' (*das Unheimliche*):

> *The projection of inner perceptions to the outside* is a primi-tive mechanism which, for instance, also influences our sense perceptions, so that it normally has the greatest share in shaping our outer world. Under conditions that have not yet been sufficiently determined even inner percep-tions of ideational and emotional processes are projected outwardly, like sense perceptions, and are used to shape the outer world, whereas they ought to remain in the *inner* world . . . Only with the development of the language of abstract thought through the association of sensory

remnants of word representations with inner processes, did the latter gradually become capable of perception. Before this took place primitive man had developed a picture of the outer world *through the outward projection of inner perceptions*, which we, with our reinforced conscious perception, must now translate back into psychology.[17]

Freud writes on the assumption that things in the world can never (actually, as such, in themselves) *be* uncanny. If they nevertheless appear uncanny to *us*, it must be because of us, not because of the objects. Our 'inner perceptions' throw a veil of emotional colouring upon naked physical reality, and it is the task of psychology to take up *the veil* and inspect *it*. Unlike Freud, for whom a would-be scientific approach was self-evident, I would nevertheless like to be bloody-minded at this point. I would ask exactly why it is that things supposedly cannot be uncanny in themselves. After all, isn't it so that we react to them with fear *because* they are uncanny? I already know Freud's answer: he would have said that we project our fears onto objects. But that is, of course, something he *must* say, if only because he has already made up his mind about what kinds of qualities can possibly belong to 'things in themselves'. To put my objection in a less provocative way, we need to ask what exactly is *meant* by saying that something is, or is not, a quality of things themselves. What is the kind of contrast we want to make, and how are our answers modified depending on the kinds of interest we have in the question?

Dirt is *sui generis*

Both anthropological and hygienic forms of reductionism derive a large part of their rhetorical powers from the association between dirt and disgust. Disgust is a reaction, and to find a thing disgusting is roughly to say that one would react to it with disgust – or perhaps that disgust is the proper or recommended reaction. On the whole, what we find disgusting is quite simply what provokes our disgust. For this reason, what I find disgusting often tells you more about me than about the things I single out in this way. Conversely, if I have explained to you why I find a thing to *be* disgusting there is no need for me to produce an additional explanation of why I am *disgusted*. An explanation would only be needed if for some reason I failed to react with disgust to something I have just described as disgusting.

In contrast, what I find to be dirty cannot be read off from my reactions of disgust. This is first of all because disgust is by no means the only or even dominant human reaction to dirt. A car engine is frequently dirty but seldom disgusting. Children at play may be very dirty without being disgusting at all. Conversely, spoiled food may be disgusting but not necessarily dirty – even though it might of course soil other things exactly in the same way as fresh food might. Secondly, and even more to the point, if I want to justify my reaction I will refer to my initial factual judgement that the item is dirty. Thus my reaction is explained in terms of the judgement rather than my judgement being explained by the reaction.

You might find it utterly uninformative to be told that dirt is dirt and not something else; yet we have seen now that there is need even for such a truism.

PART II

'DIRTY' AND 'FORBIDDEN': ANTHROPOLOGICAL REDUCTIONISM AND ITS LIMITS

One must start out with error and convert it into truth. That is, one must reveal the source of error, otherwise hearing the truth won't do any good. The truth cannot force its way in when something else is occupying its place. To convince someone of the truth, it is not enough to state it, but rather one must find the *path* from error to truth.

Wittgenstein, 'Remarks on Frazer's *Golden Bough*'[1]

FIVE

Ritual, Disorder and Pollution

Purity and danger

'How does refuse become unclean?' That is the pivotal question of contemporary theoretical treatments of dirt. This is very much due to the pioneering work of Mary Douglas in her now classical *Purity and Danger* (1966). Surveying the literature on dirt and pollution today, I honestly believe it would be easier to enumerate works that do not cite Douglas than those that do, even if the reason for citing may sometimes be that she just so obviously *must* be included in one's list of references. Her book, with the subtitle *An Analysis of Concepts of Pollution and Taboo*, was an effort to bring conceptions of soiling and pollution under the general cultural categories of order and disorder. If the question is how refuse *becomes* unclean, the implication must be that refuse is not unclean to start with but becomes so in a culturally determined defining process.

For Douglas, the definition of soiling is a matter of drawing a ritual limit between the acceptable and the prohibited. To understand the main principles of this demarcating procedure, it is perhaps best to look at her most frequently cited example: shoes on the floor and shoes on a dining table.[1] The same person may think of the same shoes as clean on the one occasion and dirty on the other. Douglas argues that the process through which a thing is defined as *unclean* essentially consists in imposing prohibitions: not to eat, not to touch, not to blend the one kind of thing with the other. Things that belong to the floor must not be placed on a table and outdoors things must not be left lying indoors.

In order to recognize soiling it is not enough to stare blindly at the object itself, but one needs comprehensive understanding of the culturally defined situation.

In her general approach to ideas of pollution and order, Douglas continues a line of thought originating in Émile Durkheim's (1858–1917) classical analysis of the concept of the holy (*le sacré*). According to Durkheim, the idea of the sacred or holy was the defining principle of life in all human communities. The holy is not reducible to the merely strange or unexplained but involves an attitude that completely differs from the profane.[2] For instance, there is nothing in natural disorders and accidents as such to mark them out as sacred as opposed to merely surprising and unusual. The distinction between the holy and the profane is, according to Durkheim, universal. Nowhere else in the history of human mind have there been two categories so radically distinct. Holiness is not a quality of any particular being or thing as such, which is also demonstrated by the fact that very different objects can count as holy in different societies. In the last analysis, feelings of reverence towards sacred objects owe their existence to relations between *human beings*, not to relations between man and the physical environment. The essence of holiness lies in the existence of a socially sanctioned system of prohibitions by means of which holy things are set apart from others. The substance of the prohibition may be quite arbitrary: sometimes it is forbidden to eat of the totem animal and sometimes the animal must be eaten, but always according to strictly defined rules. Prohibition and taboo mark the boundaries between the profane and the holy, regulating the engagement with the holy and thereby structuring life for members of the community.[3]

If, then, Durkheim was convinced that all holiness could be traced to a shared root of collectively imposed prohibitions, Douglas followed the same track in her analysis of pollution taboos. By classifying an element as clean or unclean we above all bring symbolic order to the world. 'Punishments, moral pressures, rules about not touching and not eating, a firm ritual framework, all these can do something to bring man into harmony with the rest of being.'[4]

Paraphrasing Douglas, the human being has a need quite generally to see the world as an organized whole, a unitary system with preordained places for herself, for other human beings and for material objects. Each culture develops characteristic patterns, ways of coming to terms with the contingencies of life both in thinking and in practical life. These patterns manifest themselves at large, as in social stratification, and in detail, as in ideas of cleanliness. The ideas of purity current in a culture are aspects of a general conception of order particular to that culture; they are another facet of *social* order.[5] Natural objects and their qualities enter the picture only as focal points for socially imposed rules of conduct. These cultural patterns are created and sustained by means of demarcation lines – between the familiar and the alien, the accepted and the prohibited, the clean and the unclean. Clean and unclean are an aspect of the given culture and its conceptions of order, which is also made visible in the behaviour prescribed for each social group. Different places are assigned to men, women and children; to my children and the neighbour's brats; to the healthy and the ill, to gentlemen and peasants, the living and the dead. Or consider various ways in which nature, dead or living, can be pigeonholed: earth, water, air, fire; humans, animals and plants; foodstuffs, blood, excrement. Last but not least, the relations between the sexes are perhaps the most obvious example of how conceptions of purity regulate human intercourse. In several cultures, women and, in some cases, men are defined as unclean during menstruation, after childbirth and after sexual intercourse, which results in restrictions with regard to their participation in religious (and consequently, communal) life.

Douglas presents a fascinating approach: in her view, dirt is never an isolated phenomenon but always belongs to a pattern, carried through the entire web of the given culture and highlighting its specific world view. The same basic patterns are discernible both at large, as in group relations between castes, estates or social classes, and at the micro level of customs connected with eating and cleaning. 'Where there is dirt there is system.'[6]

There is a certain ambiguity in this account. Dirt or impurity, which for Douglas may take the form of 'different kinds of impossibilities, anomalies, bad mixings and abominations,'[7] is defined as something that fails to fit into an assumed order. Here it seems that Douglas wants to come to grips with the unclean with the help of two metaphors with partly opposing tendencies: *disorder* and *otherness*. For her, the unclean element is understood as disturbing and dangerous either because it *deviates from its own place* in an order or because it, as an alien element, *has no place* in an assumed order of things. Shoes on the dining-room table would be an instance of the first kind of disturbance. They are not dirty in themselves, but unwanted in a particular place. The second kind of disturbance is exemplified by the various 'unclean animals' that have a prominent place in the argument of *Purity and Danger*. Unclean animals are impure wherever they are found, and in this sense their impurity is *absolute* for the culture that stands for the classification.

Suppression of disorder

For Douglas, dirt presupposes a stable order but it is an element with no legitimate place within the order: 'Dirt [is] created by the differentiating activity of the mind, it [is] a by-product of the creation of order.'[8] With this view, she consciously connects with Jean-Paul Sartre and refers to the Africans she has studied as 'primitive existentialists'.[9] The Lele (whose rituals she describes) 'recognize something of the fortuitous and conventional nature of the categories in whose mould they have their experience,'[10] thus giving life to the Existentialist thesis that existence precedes essence and the truth that 'the facts of existence are a chaotic jumble'.[11]

Something of the same sense of an underlying menace, the threat of the disintegration of experience, is expressed in the inner life of Antoine Roquentin, the protagonist of Sartre's *Nausea* (1938).[12] Disgusted by the respectable and mindless petits bourgeois of his environment, he perceives them merely as ridiculous and uncanny puppets as they strut about their Sunday walks in the provincial town where he finds himself stranded. People at the café appear to Roquentin as disjointed pieces of skin and flesh, while trees, bushes and pebbles in the park strike him as an undifferentiated mass of matter. In the famous 'park episode', matter itself is revealed as pure extension, a terrifying amorphous substance beyond all conventional description. This kind of existential dread is, however, necessarily a transient state of mind. For it appears that, at least for Douglas, we have no choice in the end but on the whole to continue our puppet-like bourgeois existence. Except for short flashes of time, we just *cannot* face the chaos of reality, the 'inherently untidy experience'.[13]

In such existential contexts the unclean arises in the form of non-classifiable, formless leftovers of existence – elements that cannot be pigeonholed in the readymade categories of the intellect. Dirt becomes the unsavoury reminder of the gap between the world as we would like it, neat and tidy, and its real state of disorder. And even though the details of our inherited conceptual straitjackets are historically contingent, in the end we cannot live without them, for we 'can't have all the world a jelly'.[14] Which, however, does not prevent us from periodically casting our conceptual categories aside in intoxication, laughter and aesthetic or religious ecstasy.[15] Consequently, several cultures have developed techniques for 'tear[ing] away even the veils imposed by the necessities of thought and to look at reality direct'.[16] Sexual intercourse might also be included here: the partners are without fail brought in contact with the other's body secretions and they experience the blurring of boundaries between self and other.

As already hinted, *Purity and Danger* has thoroughly influenced the Western psyche. It has been searched for arguments against xenophobia, compulsive orderliness, conventionality, male chauvinism and generally square thinking.[17] At first sight it may be surprising that a scholarly book on ritual purity – an abstruse third-world subject in the 1960s and '70s – would achieve such results. The real reason no doubt was (and is) the fact that Douglas set her sights on humanity as a whole, assuring us that modern Western cleanliness is also thoroughly ritualistic.[18] A direct line of shared ideas goes from the family spring cleaning back to the ritual purity of ancient Hebrews, and from our mental tendency to 'long for hard lines and clear concepts' to open or latent anti-Semitism.[19]

Dirt as matter out of place

For Douglas, then, dirt is 'matter out of place'. What and where the *right* place is, is defined by the symbolic system: 'If we can abstract pathogenicity and hygiene from our notion of dirt, we are left with the old definition of dirt as matter out of place.'[20] Objects we would normally hardly take notice of may suddenly appear problematic. This happens at the moment when their normal placement is disturbed – which takes us to the *locus classicus* of contemporary theories of dirt and pollution:

> Shoes are not dirty in themselves, but it is dirty to place them on the dining-table; food is not dirty in itself, but it is dirty to leave cooking utensils in the bedroom, or food bespattered on clothing; similarly, bathroom equipment in the drawing-room; clothing lying on chairs; out-door things in-doors; upstairs things downstairs; under-clothing where over-clothing should be; and so on. In short, our pollution behaviour is the reaction which condemns any object or idea likely to confuse or contradict cherished classifications.[21]

Douglas argues here that soiling consists in a form of confusion of elements from different classes, which not only implies that cleanliness involves the prevention of improper contact between incompatible categories of objects, but brings us back to the central insight that nothing is clean or dirty in itself, and everything depends on context. But does this also indicate, as Douglas would have it, that dirt is a form of disorder?

Let us look at the facts once more. Most of the illustrations in the quoted passage are certainly examples of disorder: of things and materials placed where they do not belong. But only one example (food bespattered on clothing) is an obvious case of soiling, and exactly here the description 'disorder' seems less than compelling. The other examples imply an environment that is not so much dirty as it is *messy.* We are told of shoes left on a dining table and we easily assent to the description of them as dirty. But in the end this is just because we tend to think of *dirty* shoes and not of new shoes straight out of the box. And it is even less plausible to claim that the shoes themselves are *dirt* (not just *dirty*), even though they conform to the proposed definition of 'dirt' as 'matter out of place'.

It is interesting to note that Douglas, who is generally alive to nuances and conceptual distinctions, for some reason simply ignores differences between various forms of displacement. The explanation lies in her strong commitment to the thesis that dirt is disorder. Distinctions between particular cases are simply blurred and *dirt* is allowed a free ride on the shoulders of *mess* and *untidiness.* Surely no one will deny that mess and untidiness involve disorder or lack of order, but the connection between dirt and disorder is less evident. To tidy up a room is not necessarily to clean it, and things can be cleaned without changing the way they are (dis) ordered. The phrase 'matter out of place' invites us to smooth over these distinctions. Read literally, it would be synonymous with '*misplaced* matter', which is, in many cases, a distinctly bad description of dirt. The less literal reading of 'out of place' as merely 'offending' or 'improper' is, on the other hand, not directly wrong, but it no longer conveys the idea of disorder.[22] After all, there is a complete class of objects and sites created as *legitimate* places for dirt: consider handkerchiefs, dishcloths and dustbins. Indeed, where else should remnants of food stay after a meal if not on the plate and then in the rubbish bin – instead of being swept to the floor or the tablecloth? Some places are the *right* places for dirt, and this is an integral, not only accidental, feature of many cleaning practices:

> There's a home for everything –
> Please use the bins provided.[23]

Leftovers in the dustbin certainly count as unwanted matter. But does out-of-placeness in *this* sense imply something more than just that dirt is *dirty*?

Things and stuffs may be out of place because they disturb a specific process or activity. Grime in the spark plug constitutes impurity because it disturbs the smooth functioning of a motor, which, on the other hand, does not imply that all disturbing substances are classified as *dirt*. Water in the petrol tank is also a kind of impurity but it does not count as dirt. Conversely, while a stain of gravy on my shirt certainly might have a disturbing effect on my conversation with guests, *that* is not why it counts as dirt. On the contrary, it disturbs me *because* I already know what it is: dirt. In brief, we have not yet arrived at any informative formulation of the idea that dirt is matter out of place. So far it seems to boil down to the tautologous assertion that dirt is dirty.

In spite of such circularity, the definition of dirt as matter out of place is perhaps not completely pointless. That would only be the case if the aim was to *reduce* soiling to out-of-placeness or to *explain* our reactions to soiling in terms of out-of-placeness – or perhaps, to work out a definition of 'dirt' that would allow someone with no understanding of the concept at all correctly to pick out cases of soiling. But a definition may also have the advantage of linking our attention to connections between things we already know but which we perhaps tend to overlook. Defining dirt, in a very general sense, as matter out of place at least highlights the fact that our general attitude towards dirt involves rejection. My objection to Douglas is then simply that out-of-placeness is not an *explanation* of why we reject certain materials as 'dirt'; it is only a reformulation of that rejection.

Impurity as anomaly and ambiguity

Douglas is using 'impurity' as a kind of umbrella concept for all manner of dirt, soiling, disorder, mess, confusion, abomination, danger and taboo. Sometimes her examples concern dirt in an everyday sense, sometimes they concern some offending or confusing element, sometimes ritual pollution and sometimes elements that appear dangerous or alien in some way or other.

Thus there is some ambiguity in how Douglas treats impurity. On the one hand, she hopes to demonstrate the context dependence of judgements about soiling. Food bespattered on clothing is a good example of this. Neither food, considered as nourishment, nor the garment as such is objectionable, but their improper combination makes them so. On the other hand, the ritual purity of the Old Testament is a completely different kind of case. In that text, certain animals are classified as unclean and rejected *regardless of context*. This is also the case of certain other beings noted by Douglas either in the Bible or elsewhere, including the insane, the dead, the body of a slain enemy, monstrous births and twin births.[24] Even though the biblical abominations and other examples of this kind presuppose a cultural context, they are nevertheless context-free in the sense that, within the given culture, they imply the idea of impurity as something *absolute*.

Douglas argues that these cases can also be brought under the wide umbrella of disorder. Her general thesis is that beings classified as ritually unclean have this status because of their ambiguous position between classes, which implies challenge to order.

Consider the most well-known of the Mosaic dietary rules: the avoidance of pork, now observed by Jews, Muslims and a plethora of Christian groups. Douglas argues convincingly that medical arguments, such as those appealing to the presence of the trichiniasis worm in pork (discovered only in 1828), cannot account for the practice, for whatever knowledge (if any) there may once have been about the health effects of pork, it was not transmitted to the existing religious tradition.[25] The prohibition was rather based on ideas of ritual purity, whereby various animals were assigned particular roles in a symbolic order. In Mosaic Law, the argument (if that is the word) for the impurity of the pig is as follows. Unlike oxen and sheep, which 'chew the cud' *and* are 'cloven-footed', swine 'is cloven-footed but does not chew the cud'.[26] For the opposite reason, the hare, too, was forbidden food: it 'chews the cud but does not part the hoof'.[27]

A modern reader is likely to wonder *why* these presumed facts should give rise to dietary restrictions. Douglas points out that the underlying reasoning owes its force to the nomadic background of the ancient Hebrews, a form of life that the Mosaic Law aimed both to record and to conserve. In the pastoral form of life, an almost symbiotic bond existed between man and cattle so that, unlike wild beasts, humans and their livestock belonged together. This motivated the division of non-human mammals into two main classes: cloven hoofed, ruminating ungulates and all others.[28] Deer, antelopes and similar game were allowed as food because of their close resemblance to oxen and sheep. But the division was particularly problematic with the wild boar and the hare, each fulfilling the one but not the other condition of 'pure' meat. Douglas argues that the swine and the hare were regarded as unclean because they confused the limit between the two main classes of mammals. She then suggests that the same principle is applicable to other classes of forbidden animals, offering the general conclusion: 'in general the underlying principle of cleanness in animals is that they shall conform fully to their class. Those species are unclean which are imperfect members of their class, or whose class itself confounds the general scheme of the world.'[29]

The facts of the case

Douglas also applies her theory to the other unclean animals of the Mosaic Law. She identifies the paramount principle of classification in terms of the animal's means of propulsion. According to this principle, for instance, the bat will be unclean because it is a mammal and yet winged like a bird. Following the same principle, proper fish move in the water with the help of fins, whereas eels, lampreys and shellfish break this rule and come across as deviant, and hence impure, members of the class of aquatic beings.[30] Just as human excreta cross the boundaries between self and other, thus challenging man's bodily integrity, unclean animals challenge the integrity of biological categories that uphold the intelligible world order. For Douglas, biblical abomination rules are an example of something she believes to be a general phenomenon across cultures, rooted in an inherent tendency of the human mind. But she is particularly insistent in her discussion of the Mosaic Law. I nevertheless feel we need to go back to the sources and to see exactly how much we should keep of her theory. Leviticus 11 says:

> Speak to the people of Israel, saying: From among all the land animals, these are the creatures that you may eat. Any animal that has divided hoofs and is cleft-footed and chews the cud – such you may eat. But among those that chew the cud or have divided hoofs, you shall not eat the following: the camel, for even though it chews the cud, it does not have divided hoofs; it is unclean for you. The rock badger, for even though it chews the cud, it does not have divided hoofs; it is unclean for you. The hare, for even though it chews the cud, it does not have divided hoofs; it is unclean for you. The pig, for even though it has divided hoofs and is cleft-footed, it does not chew the cud; it is unclean for you. *Of their flesh you shall not eat, and their carcasses you shall not touch; they are unclean for you.*[31]

After these verses follows a list of forbidden fish, fowl and insects, after which the prohibition of unclean hoofed animals is repeated. The focus then moves on, in 11:27, to other four-legged animals:

Every animal that has divided hoofs but is not cleft-footed or does not chew the cud is unclean for you; *everyone who touches one of them shall be unclean*. All that walk on their paws, among the animals that walk on all fours, are unclean for you; *whoever touches the carcass of any of them shall be unclean until the evening, and the one who carries the carcass shall wash his clothes and be unclean until the evening; they are unclean for you*.[32]

I have italicized parts of the biblical passages in order to highlight a kind of rhythm that rules the composition. After each specification of a major class of animals, the steadily growing list comes to a temporary halt, and instructions in the eventuality of contamination are inserted. Thus, for instance, instructions are inserted above in 11:27–8, after the definition of the class of animals with paws. The same happens below in 11:31–2 after a list of 'swarming things':

These are unclean for you among the creatures that swarm upon the earth: the weasel, the mouse, the great lizard according to its kind, the gecko, the land crocodile, the lizard, the sand lizard, and the chameleon. *These are unclean for you among all that swarm; whoever touches one of them when they are dead shall be unclean until the evening. And anything upon which any of them falls when they are dead shall be unclean, whether an article of wood or cloth or skin or sacking, any article that is used for any purpose; it shall be dipped into water, and it shall be unclean until the evening, and then it shall be clean*.[33]

The point about composition and rhythm will in fact be of importance for interpretative purposes. The question it helps us answer is: exactly what are the different animal categories here? The Mosaic Law quite obviously aspires to cover *all* possible groups of animals. For this reason, it would certainly be odd if it had nothing to say about the dog, man's close companion and an animal that counts as unclean everywhere in the Middle East. And indeed, even though the dog does not receive explicit mention, it clearly belongs to that large class of four-footed animals who 'walk on their paws' (Leviticus 11:27) – a category defined as unclean *in its entirety*. For Douglas, however, this should indicate a problem. Her theory says that uncleanness is ascribed to borderline cases, and it says the reason lies precisely in their borderline position. But now we have in our hands an entire, large and thoroughly familiar class of animals (animals with paws), all described as ritually unclean. Nor are there any reasons in Leviticus to think of this group as posing a challenge to the world order as a whole.

Douglas seems quite unaware of having run into a problem, or she perhaps deliberately confuses the issue. She assimilates animals with paws, described in Leviticus 11:27, with the immediately fol-lowing category of beings that 'swarm upon the earth' in Leviticus 11:29–30. At this point, she resorts to the King James Bible, which uses the word 'hands' instead of 'paws' in 11:27. Douglas contends that ritual uncleanness is in this verse ascribed *not* to cats and dogs, but rather to 'any creature which has *two legs and two hands* and which goes on all fours', including the mole, 'whose forefeet are uncannily hand-like'.[34]

It seems to me, however, that we have good reason not to go along with Douglas on this point; we should instead read the beginning of Leviticus 11:29 as the introduction of an entirely new group of animals. The previous verse (28 and end of 27) offers instructions concerning contamination, thus closing the preceding prohibition against animals with paws. In 29, the fresh category of small, crawling animals (*some* of which are singled out as defiling) is introduced, but nothing is now said about either hands or paws. My proposed reading is also in harmony with the existing Jewish tradition which treats cats, dogs and other animals with paws without exception as inedible; *Encyclopedia Judaica* includes all carnivores in this group.[35] Animals with paws are not borderline cases but *true* members of a well-defined class of their own, defined as impure in its entirety. Douglas is simply wrong in claiming that the main motive for the Mosaic rejection of these animals as unclean lies in any ambiguous status they might have.

To be sure, certain animal species, including the swine and the hare, receive special attention in the Mosaic dietary law; and it is quite plausible that they are thus singled out precisely because of their borderline status. Borderlines are of course places where believers would be easily tempted by creative applications of the law; it is especially important to be explicit here about where the boundaries go. This is, however, not to say that hares and pigs are *more* unclean than the more obvious members of the unclean classes, but only that one needs to be on one's guard.

One might imagine still one way to rescue the hypothesis that Douglas advocates. Suppose it is argued that whole animal classes can be rejected because the entire class may be seen as a borderline case. Douglas makes this attempt vis-à-vis 'swarming things'. As a form of movement, she says, 'swarming' (also translatable as teeming, crawling and so on) is 'an indeterminate form of movement' – 'not a mode of propulsion proper to any particular element', hence it 'cuts across the basic classification. Swarming things are neither fish, flesh nor fowl'.[36] Douglas suggests that this class of beings straddles the earth–sky–water division, marking them out as beings that challenge the natural order of creation. These claims by Douglas invite, first of all, this response. The fact that 'swarming' animals are not acceptable members of the *other* classes by no means justifies calling them borderline cases; on the contrary it is precisely a good reason for perceiving them as a class of their own. Secondly, the quoted biblical passages speak explicitly of 'things that swarm upon the *earth*', not indicating any breach of boundaries between land, air and sea. Finally, the text does not appear to say that *all* swarming things are forbidden, and it does not state that the prohibition is on account of their form of movement.

It would of course be simple to respond with a logical point. If all that matters is what is logically non-contradictory, *any* group of entities can 'logically speaking' be construed as borderline cases. In order to do that, it is enough to settle for some dichotomy that *makes* the group stand out as borderline; if we insist that everything be black or white, any other colour will duly come out as ambiguous. But then of course the factual question remains of whether the people under scrutiny, say the ancient Hebrews, *did* think of a given animal as a borderline case. One might similarly, for instance, maintain that body secretions are borderline, for they confuse the limit between the body and the outside. Fair enough – but do we have real records of someone confusing a bit of faeces with a hand, a foot or some other part of the human body?

Douglas is somewhat ambiguous about what it means to confuse borders, or what it means for the human being to create order in the universe. In this connection, she is primarily thinking of intellectual order: to create order is to classify things, to fit them into a coherent world view. The unclean species are those which resist classification. For instance, bats are anomalous because they have an ambiguous position between birds and mammals, and lampreys are anomalous members of the class of fish, conceived as aquatic beings with scales and fins. When the projection of intellectual order meets with cases that resist obvious classification, two kinds of correcting movement will be available. *Stipulation* means that a definite border is drawn where a blurred border was earlier in place; as when, in modern biology, a certain set of biological similarities override others, and bats are defined as mammals rather than birds (this involves the additional principle that an animal cannot be a mammal and a bird *at the same time*). The other possibility, *the creation of a new class*, means that the anomalous entity is redefined as a normative member of a class of its own. This happens when biologists define lampreys as a group of their own instead of as a kind of anomalous fish. The existence of challenges to a classificatory scheme may be called intellectual disorder; however, such challenges simply point to limitations of the scheme. Order is restored through revisions of the scheme.

So far so good, but the link to our ordinary cleaning and tidying efforts now seems tenuous. To tidy up a room is to implement an existing conception of order, which normally does not involve any deep uncertainty about classification. Garments lying on the floor offend my sense of order precisely because (and only to the extent that) I *know* their proper place is not there.[37] There is no obvious positive link between untidiness and uncertain class identity. In sum, we may distinguish between three kinds of challenge to order amongst the examples that Douglas is discussing:

1. In some cases, class identity is not disputed but the item is physically displaced (cf. garments on the floor, food on clothing and shoes on the dining table).
2. For a second group of items, regardless of physical placement, class identity is ambiguous (cf. cloven-hoofed non-ruminating ungulates).
3. In yet some cases, class identity is not ambiguous, but the class as a whole is rejected (cf. enemies, excrement, animals with paws).

In her discussion of Mosaic dietary law, Douglas assimilates group (3) with group (2). Furthermore, she also describes group (1) as identical with group (2), because she does not distinguish between physical displacement and intellectual ambiguity. Given the vagueness of her central theoretical concept of 'disorder', her central thesis about the borderline character of the rejected items appears highly questionable.

Background and foreground

In her book, Douglas contributes to a respectable tradition in the social sciences that might be described as one of *revelation through relativity*. It is the tradition of unmasking hidden meanings of social institutions by seeing them not as self-evident but as dependent on culture. The social anthropologist who studies an alien society will, among other things, try to formulate the rules that its members follow in their daily lives. For instance, a culture involves a certain sense of propriety, which the anthropologist may try to convey in the form of a list of actions regarded as improper and forbidden. But it is important for what is meant by 'sense of propriety' that the locals tend to see proper behaviour not simply as implementing set rules, but as expressing a *natural* attitude characteristic of sane adults. Where the locals see natural and rational behaviour, the anthropologist – who to some extent by definition adopts the position of an outsider – will see behaviour that is everywhere circumscribed by rules.

Now suppose the anthropologist turns her gaze back to her home culture and tries to identify features in it that strike her as similar to the ones she has studied. Whatever she looks at she will now see through a relativizing prism, showing up the received world view of her own culture as merely symbolic, culturally specific and historically contingent. This perhaps accounts for some of the lay appeal of social anthropology and cultural sociology: they afford us both the necessity of cultural self-reflection and the luxury of cynicism. In assessing Douglas, we need to take account of this peculiar kind of disparity between the home perspective and the anthropological gaze. We must introduce a distinction between cultural *foreground and background*.

Anyone who lives among his or her own people will have a natural inside understanding of the cultural categories that they employ. Certain phenomena, such as the existence of unwashed dishes in the kitchen, are simply seen as facts. Relevant standards of cleanliness enter perception as a self-evident background against which further questions are raised and answered – for instance, 'Can I leave the dishes now and wash up later?' The distinction between cultural foreground and background implies, however, that what the insider treats as self-evident facts will, for the anthropologist, who works as an outsider, stand out as expressions of culturally determined *attitudes*. In the present case, objects mixed or smeared with unwanted substances must be isolated or they must be immersed in water according to custom. The outsider could formulate this as a rule which must be observed in cases of alleged pollution. In similar ways, the entire life of the alien culture appears to be circumscribed by rules, and it falls on the anthropologist to make those rules explicit to her readers.

From her resulting description of our culturally determined rules and prohibitions, the visiting anthropologist might, for example, draw the conclusion that it is *forbidden* in our culture to wear garments with bloodstains. However, while she might say we follow an unwritten rule, from our insiders' perspective we would not think of our behaviour as the result of a *prohibition* at all. We do not feel inclined to go against the alleged rule, for we feel that a clean garment is just preferable to one that is not; thus we do not perceive the issue in terms of rules but in terms of facts. To be sure, facts subsequently give rise also to prohibitions; it is, for instance, an offence to deliberately ruin someone else's clothes with blood. We also face practical questions about the best stain-removing methods. This background of facts must also be understood differently from rites and symbols. I cite Isaiah once more:

> When you stretch out your hands, I will hide my eyes from you; even though you make many prayers, I will not listen; your hands are full of blood. Wash yourselves; make yourselves clean; remove the evil of your doings from before my eyes; cease to do evil ... Come now, let us argue it out,

says the Lord: though your sins are like scarlet, they shall
be like snow; though they are red like crimson, they shall
become like wool.[38]

The prophet's comparison of sin with soiling draws its force from
a self-evident fact, the difference between dirty and clean linen, on
which its very intelligibility is based. A symbol can do work only in
a context of meaningful facts; conversely, to describe a fact as *merely*
symbolic is to dispute its independent value. The confusing identification of moral and ritual pollution with factual dirt, found in
Purity and Danger, involves confusion between a symbol and the
background conditions of its intelligibility. Now looking back to
the Old Testament, we need to recognize that neither we nor the
ancient Hebrews primarily thought of cleanliness as a *symbolic* practice. Both sin and the so-called unclean foodstuffs were treated *as if*
they involved factual soiling, but in the background of all this
loomed the undisputed facts of real, non-symbolic soiling. If someone shies away from an untidy kitchen there is nothing symbolic
about what disgusts her. Thus our concepts of dirty and clean, which
are not essentially based on prohibitions, must be kept apart from
possibly related, but typically ritual practices. The latter presuppose
the former.

In an interesting simile, philosopher Peter Winch has compared
the anthropologist not with an engineer observing the outcome of
experiments in a laboratory, but with an apprentice engineer trying
to figure out the routines of his senior colleagues.[39] Here is a way
to develop that comparison: senior engineers (the natives) operate
their machinery with a secure hand and they can immediately see
the implications of a given move. The apprentice (the anthropologist), however, needs guidance in order not to spoil the experiment
and perhaps even hurt herself. Thus the senior engineers focus on
their research question and the contribution of the experiment
towards solving it, while the apprentice concentrates on learning
the rules that obtain in the laboratory. The senior engineer will not

touch a certain machine part because that would be dangerous; the apprentice will not touch it because it is forbidden. Issuing prohibitions is, in many cases, the first stage towards teaching someone a new skill.

But it is only the *first* stage. We forbid our children to fiddle with electric sockets because it is dangerous. However, the child has understood us correctly only once it refrains not because it is forbidden but because it understands the danger of it. Similarly, the child has really understood why one should not touch dirty objects or put them in one's mouth when the child no longer thinks of the situation in terms of prohibitions. It is true that, even in adult life, we are sometimes tempted to neglect hygiene and safety, but that is not because deep down we prefer dirt and danger but because there might be other, overriding interests. It would be misleading to describe our practical cleanliness simply as a body of restrictions on behaviour. It is rather the inherited background of our other practices, built on the self-evident distinction between clean and dirty, made naturally by competent adults.

Cultural practices will, then, appear differently depending on whether we look at them from the outside or the inside. As observers and self-observers, we have some freedom of movement between the two perspectives. However, it does not appear meaningful to ask, as a general question, which of the two perspectives is the *right* one. There are certainly reasons sometimes to look at one's society at a distance, reminding oneself of the diversity of human culture; and sometimes reasons not to.

Consider, for instance, the idea of the nuclear family and the ideas of marriage associated with it. Consider further the predictable emotional conflicts that arise from the twin ideas of romantic love and life-long monogamy, conflicts that are the standard stuff of the bourgeois novel. It will be useful to consider that those tragedies were (and are) only possible in a particular kind of society, while tragedy in other societies takes other forms. The Western bourgeois family is a historically and geographically limited phenomenon not to be projected onto other times and places indiscriminately. I understand all this very well; however, it is of no help to me if I am troubled by goings-on in *my* nuclear family. The ancient Hebrews would not have had my exact problems, but then again, I am not an ancient Hebrew either. My own situation is in a sense the accidental product of a culturally and historically specific situation, but it nevertheless remains my task to figure out what to do about it. If I ask what love is – what it is to love someone – I will have (to start with, at least) to ask what love means to me, in this particular time and place. In this sense philosophical arguments are always *ad hominem*.

The role of perception

Very well – we, children of a particular time and place, perceive our environment in terms of the dirty-and-clean distinction. We seldom question it, it appears natural to us, and perhaps in some situations it cannot be helped. But might it not now be asked: what is the world really like, apart from *our* ways of perceiving? Is dirt really an element of the material world, or is it just a way for *us* to understand it? In other words: might not Douglas have a point when she argues that dirt is not so much an element of reality as the result of a symbolic order that we *impose* on reality?

At this juncture we need to reflect on perception. Douglas advances an argument that presupposes two levels. On the one level, 'out there' is reality, raw and unclassified. On the other hand, the human being – or culture – creates a second level, a system for bringing various elements of reality into meaningful relations with each other. According to Douglas, we normally encounter reality in perception only once it is filtered through this second, meaning-producing layer. What are her ideas about elementary, not-yet-humanly-classified reality *before* it passes the filter? Is it possible in the first place to describe such reality, free of the veils drawn over it by our intellectual and emotional nature?

In fact Douglas appears to count on the possibility of unmediated contact with reality.[40] Such contact, she thinks, is an exceptional experience and she refers to Sartre's feelings of existential Angst as an example.[41] However, despite her gestures towards Existentialism, it seems to me that Douglas is ultimately paying tribute to the post-Galilean cult of science. She makes use of an implicit metaphysics that denies the capacity of everyday experience to present reality as it is, and which implicitly takes natural science to be the arbiter of questions about the true character of reality. A world containing *meaningful* elements is merely a projection of human consciousness. On the other hand, despite her use of Sartre in this context, it does not seem obvious to me that this is also *Sartre's* view. In any case we should not presume, as a matter of course, that Roquentin is identical with the novelist, or that the novelist is identical with the philosopher.

Simultaneously with *Nausea*, Sartre was working on philosophical essays that address the relation between experience and reality. A thoroughgoing motif here is the idea that naive, unreflective experience does not need to be explained, supported or brought into question by material that belongs to the stage of reflection. In philosophical literature, love, hate, fear and sympathy are typically treated as emotions projected by the perceiver onto the environment, but Sartre wants to side with the pre-reflective experience that sees them as so many ways to *discover* the existing lovable, hateful, fearful and endearing qualities of things. Perhaps Sartre's most uncompromising formulations on this score are included in his brief essay on *Intentionality* from 1939. A Japanese theatre mask is not a carved piece of wood on which I project my fear; fearfulness is a quality of the mask and cannot be divorced from it. And Sartre wants to return us to 'that truth so deeply distrusted by our refined thinkers: that if we love a woman, it is because she *is lovable*'.[42] For Sartre, emotion is one of our ways to come closer to the object of perception. In contrast, Douglas describes perception as a kind of falsification:

It is generally agreed that all our impressions are schematically determined from the start. In a chaos of shifting impressions, each of us constructs a stable world in which objects have recognisable shapes, are located in depth, and have permanence . . . *Uncomfortable facts, which refuse to be fitted in, we find ourselves ignoring or distorting so that they do not disturb these established assumptions.* By and large anything we take note of is pre-selected and organized in the very act of perceiving. We share with other animals a kind of filtering mechanism which at first only lets in sensations we know how to use.[43]

Douglas argues here that we – that is, our nervous systems – construct a model of the world on the basis of sense impressions. This is a theory widely employed in the psychology of perception. However, her constructivist interpretation of the idea of pollution is somewhat ambiguous, as we can see by comparing the italicized part with the rest of the quote. If we are to *ignore* or *distort* facts we must start by perceiving them. The question is then whether dirt is a fact that we first perceive and then distort, or whether the crucial moment is to be sought at the earlier stages of perception, when the nervous system filters out anomalous signals? In the latter case *those* signals cannot constitute the unwanted experience that is ignored or distorted.[44] Hence *they* cannot constitute the anomalies that make up the category of dirt.

Now consider the other possibility: our experience of dirt consists of material that has already passed the cognitive filter, and the category of 'dirt' is to be understood as an organizing principle imposed on an originally neutral experience. 'Dirt [is] created by the differentiating activity of the mind.'[45] What now remains unclear is how to characterize the supposedly original and *neutral* experience. What is its object? Chemical stuff? Atoms? Extended matter? If we take Douglas at her word, all these descriptions should run into the same problem: they are not cognitively pristine, but they, like *any* general concept, result from the same kind of classificatory activity that assumedly gave rise to the perception of dirt.

The conclusion is: 'dirt' as a category is neither more nor less *constructed* than 'gravy' or 'carbohydrates'. If we follow up this thread a bit longer we must also conclude that, for Douglas, there simply can be no such thing as perceiving *anything* as it really is. For Douglas, this kind of general scepticism would not be good news even though her theory seems to imply it. After all, she wanted to keep the possibility of establishing a contrast between pollution, as a subjective result of human production of meaning, and an objective, *identifiable* world of tangible facts. Now it seems that 'physical objects', 'gravy' and 'dirt' all go down the same drain of 'symbolic order' – and we are left with 'all the world a jelly'.

SIX

Repressing the 'Other': The Myth of Abjection

The abject and the categories of thought

Recent theoretical work on soiling, refuse and pollution has mostly used the work of Douglas as a starting point. The central theme is how *limits* are drawn between individuals, between social groups and between nature and culture. In the last analysis, the guiding question concerns nothing less than the very conditions of possible thought and experience.

Immanuel Kant famously claimed that nature is never available to us as it is – in the form of 'the thing in itself' – but is always already in shapes that *we* read into it by virtue of the structure of our cognitive apparatus. As Kant makes clear in *The Critique of Pure Reason*, meaningful judgements about reality imply two intimately connected dimensions: on the one hand one that is *a priori*, rational and in agreement with the forms of thought given to us in logic and in *a priori* forms of intuition; on the other hand the dimension of empirical information based on perception. Regardless of what future experiences are in store for us, we already know that they will occur in a universe of linear time and three-dimensional space where the laws of cause and effect are operative.

That was Kant; but is there reason to go along with him? Where does he get his conviction that our experience and judging will forever conform to the principles he has laid out? Kant's answer is: because our thinking always presents the material from experience as *ordered*, and therefore our judgements must present themselves in terms of specific forms or categories of thought (such as the categories of possibility and impossibility, necessity and contingency, cause and effect).[1] In other words, if it is only with the help of forms of intuition and logical categories that we can think of something as existing, as a possible object of knowledge,[2] then those limiting conditions must be taken as given or *transcendental*. They are, according to Kant, ultimately expressions of just what it means for any subject to relate itself to any objective reality. To ask whether some *other* kind of thought might be possible is just as senseless as to ask whether logic must necessarily be logical.

Now suppose someone still wants to ask: what about the world in itself, independent of human cognitive capacities? What kind of a logical and experiential order does *it* have? A meaningless question, Kant would say. We cannot think beyond the limits of thought. In fact, even that way of putting it would concede too much because it suggests the image of a limit and therefore the unavoidable idea of crossing the limit and finding something on the other side. As if something *might* be done but *we*, for some reason or other, just couldn't pull it off. For Kant, 'to transcend the limits of thought' is not to think in some new, unheard-of way – but simply *not* to think.

More than a hundred years later, with Idealist philosophy on the wane, Durkheim reopened the question of the necessities of thought. 'Saying that the categories are necessary because they are indispensable to the functioning of the intellect', he protested, 'is simply repeating that they are necessary'.[3] He argued that an explanation is needed, and that it must be given in the form of a *naturalization* of our forms of intuition and thought. It must be shown that the necessities of thought can be explained as effects of human natural and social conditions. This is the suggestion developed further in contemporary philosophies of dirt. Durkheim argued that the compulsive power of categories over our thinking is, in the last instance, just an effect of the compulsive power of *social* order. Conversely, social order can only be upheld as long as the members of society agree in their ways of organizing their thought. But all of this is historically accidental; it depends on power relations, and accordingly it can be unmasked and challenged as well as transcended.

The relevance of dirt and defilement to these originally Durkheimian questions is stressed, for instance, in the work of Julia Kristeva. For Kristeva, our normal thinking makes use of culturally determined symbolic systems, which are the normal frameworks for all our questioning and answering, and which in the last analysis allow us to conceptualize the world in the shape of dichotomies – true vs false, yes vs no. However, she believes also a third alternative is possible, namely everything *not* represented in the system: everything thrown out or 'abject'. The human reaction to the excluded element is one of disgust, dread or abjection.[4] This is why our reactions to filth are philosophically important. They become a sort of experimental confirmation of the fact that some parts of reality lie outside the reach of pure and ordered thinking. Kristeva cites Douglas and other anthropological sources for documentation of a 'logic of *exclusion* that causes the abject to exist':[5]

> Because it is excluded as a possible object, asserted to be a non-object of desire, abominated as ab-ject, as abjection, filth becomes defilement and founds on the henceforth released side of the 'self and clean' the order that is thus only (and therefore, always already) sacred.[6]

In this way, the contrast between clean and dirty is ultimately assimilated to the contrast between *self* and *other*, which is at the same time the contrast between the logical and the non-logical. The logical, the self and clean, is further identified with the profane and familiar, and the non-logical with the sacred.

A few things should be obvious from the previous paragraphs. In the debate now under consideration, dirt and filth are predominantly treated as 'other', as something absolutely rejected rather than as something dependent on situational and practical considerations. Furthermore, the discussion is theory-driven in the sense that its main focus does not lie on soiling as such. Rather it is aimed at generally poking about in the backyards of civilization, looking for whatever does not quite fit into the assumed structures of social life and thought, whereby everything deviant is seized on as a potential example of 'otherness'. It will also be in place to speak of a *myth* here because, in the typical manner of a mythical idea, this conception of defilement comes into play at several cultural levels – in art, literature and political thought as well as in academic research. By calling it a myth I now reveal my own attitude. On the one hand I advise caution, on the other I believe the whole enterprise is not really a theory with truth claims, but more like a picture aimed at presenting a perspective on our place in the universe. Hence the crucial question is not, 'Is the picture a true one?' but, 'Does it clarify things or does it blur them?'

The whole enterprise must reasonably be treated as a feature of *Western* cultural self-understanding: the savage and the primitive, like the neurotic and the infant, came in handy for Europeans as mirrors in which they wished (not) to see themselves, or perhaps simply as screens on which they could project their secret desires and fears.

The holy as a limiting notion

Durkheim, a Founding Father of sociology, still beckons us at the entrance. Durkheim's sociological interest above all focused on the question of social solidarity, of what keeps a society together. This is also true of his great work on 'primitive' religion, *The Elementary Forms of the Religious Life*, first published in 1912. His main question is of universal significance. How can we explain that ordinary men and women, the individuals all societies are made of, are in some conditions prepared to sacrifice their personal welfare and even their lives for the good of society? Reasonably enough Durkheim rejects social contract theory, an idea of the origin of society that he attributes (correctly) to Hobbes and (incorrectly) to Rousseau. Social life cannot be ultimately based on any kind of contract, but on the contrary, social solidarity already implies community.[7]

In the introductory and concluding chapters of *The Elementary Forms*, Durkheim makes it clear he wants to connect the question of social solidarity with the idea of naturalizing the categories of thought (among which he, unlike Kant, also includes time and space, the forms of intuition).[8] He argues that the characteristic feature of the categories lies in the *compulsion* that they exert on thinking. They are norms about how we should think – but where do norms come from? Durkheim's answer is: they must come from society. The necessities of social organization allow nothing else:

> If men do not agree upon these essential ideas at every moment, if they did not have the same conception of time, space, cause, number, etc., all contact between their minds would be impossible, and with that, all life together. Thus society could not abandon the categories to the free choice of the individual without abandoning itself.[9]

Society is, more than anything else, kept together because its members think in the same way. Deviants are excluded and branded as lunatics or evildoers.[10] Dominant norms of thought must be presented as inviolable, and the role of religion and *the holy* will be central in the process. Religion captures Durkheim's interest because, for him, it is the meeting place for everything crucial for the relation between individual and society: external, anonymous, collective pressure on individual thinking and, as the source of this pressure, the 'collective consciousness' of the community.

For Durkheim, the holy was *heterogeneous*, literally perceived to be 'of other origin than' the profane. Prohibition and taboo would mark its boundaries, minimizing the risk of unregulated contacts over the crucial dividing line between the holy and the profane.[11] Anthropologists of Durkheim's time argued that in this respect, the holy was reminiscent of another category that one might have imagined to be its complete opposite: *the unclean*. In fact they believed that the difference could sometimes collapse altogether: an object was unclean *because* it was holy and it was holy because unclean. The main thing was simply its heterogeneity, its absolute otherness. Scholarly debate eagerly adopted this idea of *the ambivalence of the holy*. Primitive man, it was held, approached the holy with love and respect but also with loathing and fear, a sense of the uncanny. This idea was originally introduced by Robertson Smith, British theologian and anthropologist of the late nineteenth century, known for his work on early Semitic religion.[12] The ambivalence of the holy soon developed a life of its own and it has been described as an academic myth.[13] For the present purpose there is no need to assess the truth of the claim itself but only to trace its fortunes in Western intellectual discourse.

Looking back to Durkheim, it can be said he paints a mainly positive picture of the effects of social cohesion, a fact that surely contributed to his posthumous status as a kind of official ideologue for the French late Third Republic. But the following generation of scholars came to focus on exclusion, the dark side of solidarity; including, for instance, Carl Schmitt, once known as the legal theorist of the Third Reich.[14] In sum, thinkers active between the two world wars took up aspects of integration that were already implicit in Durkheim's work but not fully developed. The discussion of dirt and defilement was carried further partly by members of the Durkheim school[15] and partly by Sigmund Freud (1856–1939) during the latter part of his career. These threads meet in Georges Bataille and later in Julia Kristeva, becoming a source of inspiration for scholars today.

Taboo, obsessional neurosis and the Beast Inside

Having consolidated his psychoanalytic movement Freud made increasingly bold excursions into the domains of cultural history and social analysis. With *Totem and Taboo* (first published in 1913), followed later by *Civilization and Its Discontents* (1930) and *Moses and the Monotheistic Religion* (1938–9), he embarks on the then ongoing debate concerning the foundations of social life and morality – themes that kept his fantasy occupied in his later years.[16] Like Durkheim, he seized upon the idea of the ambivalence of the sacred. The Polynesian word *taboo* means, like *sacer*, its Latin counterpart, both 'sacred, consecrated to the gods' and 'uncanny, dangerous, forbidden, unclean'.[17] The common denominator lies according to Freud in *the prohibition to touch* as well as in the idea that holiness/ defilement is contagious and transmitted via touch. Breaking a taboo is often heavily invested with feeling. Infringements must be removed through expiatory ceremonies, ritual purification that often involves ritual washing with water.[18] This is, according to Freud, also the original meaning of the modern concept of the holy.

Since taboo has no rational explanation, how is it to be understood? The first riddle lies in what appears to be the completely arbitrary manner in which the relevant objects are set apart as forbidden. The second is the incredible strength of taboo, in spite of the fact that it rationally appears to be completely unmotivated. The third problem is ambivalence, the (assumed) fact that forbidden objects are perceived as both fascinating and repulsive at the same time.

The solution, a constant motif in Freud's cultural analysis – something of a master key for him – is the assumed parallel between personal and cultural development. Psychologically, the maturation of each individual proceeds through the very stages that once marked human progress from animal existence to civilization. That the global South would represent the childhood of humankind was accepted as self-evident in the anthropology of the time (and was of course a cornerstone of colonial expansion).

It is, for instance, implicit in the influential volumes by Sir James Frazer from which Freud gathered most of his information about 'savages' or 'primitive races'. Now if savages were children, nothing was more natural than making inverted use of the original idea: material from childhood development might be correspondingly made to throw light on primitive culture. But Freud's contention was furthermore that neurotics represented arrested development on the road from infancy to adulthood – the main point being 'the psychological correspondence between taboo and compulsion neurosis'.[19] Hence the subtitle of *Totem and Taboo*: *Resemblances Between the Psychic Lives of Savages and Neurotics*.

Infant, neurotic and savage minds are characterized by magical thinking. It operates with symbolic connections while real causal influences are ignored – thus magic assumes the 'Omnipotence of Thought', the ability to change the world through mere imagination.[20] Relations between ideas are mistaken for relations between things. In compulsive or obsessional neurosis, steadily new objects assume a threatening character because thinking creates chains of association between the objects and the patient's fears. Freud, applying a classification made popular by Frazer, argues that two magical principles are operative here.[21] In *contagious* magic, qualities and forces are transmitted from one object to another via physical contact (the hand that touches the forbidden object becomes itself ceremonially unclean), while the principle of *imitative* or homeopathic magic implies influences between objects that resemble each other (one may try to injure an enemy by producing an effigy and mutilating it).

Freud includes in his work several examples of parallelism between taboo and the avoidance of dirt. In both cases, pollution is transmitted via physical contact, and the prohibition to touch is the central element. Breaking rules about touching gives rise to a sense of unease and the longing for purification. In *Totem and Taboo*, however, Freud is careful to distinguish between ritual defilement and factual soiling. The former is ultimately an expression of the prohibition against incest while avoidance of the latter may quite simply serve 'aesthetic and hygienic purposes'.[22] In fact, this distinction is fundamental for Freud's project at this stage, because the central difference between the sane adult, that is, you and me, and the infant, the neurotic and the savage is said to lie precisely in the fact that we, unlike them, can perceive the difference between reality and symbol. To be sure, the basic distinction between the magic of defilement and practical hygiene is compatible with sometimes using real hygiene as a symbol, as with Pontius Pilate, or as in the example that Freud cites from Frazer: he speaks of 'the warriors of a savage tribe' imposing 'the greatest chastity and cleanliness upon themselves as soon as they go upon the war-path'.[23] Freud even counts on the possibility that 'magic motivations' may be employed to 'cover', mask or hide (drapieren) aesthetic and practical considerations.[24] Nevertheless a firm difference between symbol and reality is assumed.

In Freud's later book Civilization and Its Discontents[25] this basic distinction is, however, crumbling. Now cleaning and tidying efforts appear altogether symbolic also among Europeans. Freud is simply losing faith in civilization, for we are all savages and our form of life is neurotic. The forever rising hygienic standards typical of civilized society, of no obvious utility either for biological survival or for the general quality of life, are simply obsessive, even if they are rationalized and masked by health considerations (whereas in Totem and Taboo Freud had still been talking of 'masking' in the opposite sense).[26]

If then our obsession with cleanliness pre-exists any knowledge of possible health effects, and if its roots are symbolic rather than factual, then its origins must be sought in childhood development – more precisely, in toilet training. We see the wizard once more reaching for his master key, which is now more and more assuming the look of a crowbar. Freud argues that the development of the individual child is only a replay of the collective prehistory of humankind: one must assume 'equivalence between the cultural process and the libidinous development of the individual'.[27] In toilet training, the infant is taught to feel disgust towards its own excrement, which it initially perceives as a valuable, detached part of its own body, whereby the basic distinction between the self and the external world is established. In going through this development, the infant ultimately re-enacts the decisive moment when the human species learned to walk erect, freeing the hands and the faculty of sight for the rational manipulation of surrounding objects. Dirt stands proxy for faeces and for the infantile desire to revert to a state of nature, an existence dominated by olfaction. Toilet training prohibits every manner of relapse into animal life forms.

> Such re-evaluation would hardly be possible unless this matter extracted from the body were doomed, due to its strong odour, to participate in the general fate reserved for olfactory stimuli after man learned to walk erect and left the earth surface. Anal eroticism, then, became the first victim of the 'organic repression' that prepared the way for culture.[28]

Freud was typically not too explicit about his debt to philosophical predecessors, perhaps because he liked to think of himself as an empirical scientist, not as a speculative thinker. It is in any case not far-fetched to think he was influenced by Kant's brief essay on the 'Presumable Beginnings of Human History'.[29] For Kant, what makes us human is the exercise of self-restraint (Kant would hardly be Kant otherwise). Man's original fall from grace or transition from animal to human existence meant that he refrained from acting on mere impulse and gave pride of place to reason. Kant connects this with the hegemony of sight over smell. The olfactory and gustatory senses operate on the simple evaluative axis of delicious to disgusting, while the sense of sight allows for a *discursive* response. Emotive responses to objects of sight almost always build on the previous *identification* of what is seen. The primacy of the eye over the nose and the mouth lie at the root of rational thought.

In contrast it appears however that, for Freud, the average European was not ruled by reason. We have certainly brought our animal impulses under control, but in exchange we let ourselves be guided by magical thinking. Nevertheless Freud was not dismissive of Western rationality as such, for he continued to see the control of affects as a generally positive thing, despite the price we have to pay in the form of civilization and its discontents – the repression of instinct through the Superego, requiring that we renounce everything animal and therefore everything impure and dirty. The next generation after Freud was not so sure.

The heterogeneous as the limit of meaning

We now consider Georges Bataille (1897–1962), who worked with similar anthropological material to Durkheim and Freud, becoming a precursor of what later was to be known as poststructuralism. Perhaps he has even stimulated research in the humanities as a whole: for instance, historians have now, just as he hoped, understood the relevance of research in social margins and the marginalized groups of society.[30] For the most part it is difficult to state exactly where new ideas come from, because very similar thoughts often seem to occur to many people at once when the intellectual atmosphere is right. In the case of Bataille, the situation is even worse because his constant return to the themes of disgust and sadism may have caused scholars both to underplay and to exaggerate his influence. As to his own background, the influence of the Durkheim school is obvious.

In the manner of Durkheim, Bataille believed that the limits of possible thought (the necessity of the categories) must be viewed in the context of social stratification and exclusion, including both the expulsion of social outsiders as 'others' and the drawing of limits between clean and unclean. Both, he submits, involve *excretion* of unwanted elements from the system, to be studied more exactly in a projected field of research by the name of 'Heterology' or 'Scatology' – the study of the other, the study of faeces.[31] Bataille conceives of the homogeneous and the heterogeneous as the two basic categories of human existence, tracing their roots to the twin impulses of *appropriation* and *excretion*.[32] The homogeneous is the 'own' and familiar, clean and discursively intelligible; the heterogeneous is the 'other' and alien, the defiled and defiling, the unsayable and unthinkable which, in accordance with the principle of ambivalence, may be both unclean and holy at the same time.

By this, Bataille believed he was able to explain why our culture assigns not only excrement, refuse and vermin to the sphere of heterogeneous, but also 'body parts, persons, words and deeds of erotic significance' as well as non-homogeneous social groups like 'the masses, the classes of warriors, aristocrats and the poor, different kinds of violent individuals or individuals who at least refuse to conform (lunatics, leaders, poets etc.)'.[33]

When an element comes out as heterogeneous, it is always *with regard to* some principle of organization – for instance, familiarity, value, practicability or usefulness. The heterogeneous is whatever contrasts with the principle as the 'other' to it, which implies that no object is heterogeneous as such and in itself; and so it could not be stated, for instance, that faeces are always heterogeneous. To study human excrement directly is already to bring it into a discursive universe, but the heterogeneous is the absolute Other. To define it and describe it is already to lose sight of its otherness. Our understanding can close in on the heterogeneous only in an indirect way. Heterology can, however, hope to describe human ways of *relating to* otherness, which for Bataille include on the one hand the processes of excretion and exclusion and on the other the sense of simultaneous repulsion and attraction exercised by the rejected elements.[34] As to the *subjective* heterogeneity of specific materials – for instance of the juices of a decaying, decomposing corpse – it can be felt directly in experience.[35] Heterogeneity can also take a religious or erotic form or it may be felt as dread.

The limits of the homogeneous are explored and demonstrated in part by studying the interfaces and in part by means of experimental *transgression*, in momentary carnivals of ecstasy, absurdity, crime, sadism, intoxication, of letting oneself go. This is also explored in the series of lectures that Bataille held in 1951–3 on the topic of non-knowledge (*non-savoir*), describing laughter and sobbing as examples of heterogeneous experience.[36]

Strictly speaking there is nothing in the idea of heterology as such to imply value judgement over the cultural process of excretion. Indeed such judgements would seem to be meaningless from the start, for they would have to be made from the inside of the very discourse that is judged. Nevertheless Bataille gives us quite clear signals. The heterogeneous stands for the creative, for what giveth life; the homogeneous stands for the letter that killeth.[37] Modern humanity leads a life devoid of any preordained meaning. Life's complexities and ambiguities are due to the fact that it consists of both what is intelligible and what is unintelligible, each being a constitutive part of it. 'Evil' equals the unintelligible and uncontrollable, death being its chief instance. But if death is implied in life as its constitutive limit, then 'evil' is a condition of 'good'. Confronting death gives life intensity and meaning. Consequently, meaning is not identical with the good. Meaning is created *within* life by *consciously willing the uncontrollable*.[38] As an example, Bataille refers to *potlatch*, the feast among Native North Americans of the Pacific coast where property is systematically destroyed.[39] He sums up his theoretical ambitions in this way:

> Above all, Heterology is opposed to any manner of homogeneous representation of the world, that is, to any philosophical system. Such representations always aim at depriving the universe as far as possible of any source of excitement and at developing a servile human space, merely fit for the purposes of the manufacture, rational consumption and conservation of products. But the intellectual

process automatically limits itself by creating its own waste products, thus liberating the heterogeneous element of excrement in a disorganized way. Heterology simply takes up consciously and resolutely this terminal process, which up to this point has been seen as the miscarriage and shame of human thought. *It is precisely here that it* [Heterology] *goes about in complete reversal of the philosophical process – as it turns, from being an instrument of appropriation, to the service of excretion, reclaiming the violent forms of satisfaction implicit in social life.*[40]

Kant's idea was that there are definite limits to what may be known. The implication was that the aim of philosophy lies in clarifying the logical order that lies on the familiar, meaningful side of the limits of thought and language. Bataille's aim is obviously different: he wants to transcend the limits and, in an act of Dionysian ecstasy, get hold of something alien and unsayable.

Julia Kristeva and abjection

Julia Kristeva is probably the most famous dirt theorist currently living. The publication of her *Pouvoirs de l'horreur* in English (as *Powers of Horror*) in 1982 inaugurated a stream of theoretical work on 'abject studies' and a new high of 'abject art' in galleries.[41] In her work Kristeva goes back to Durkheim, Freud, Bataille and Douglas. She takes over the Freudian foundation myth of the slaying of the primeval father as the beginning of the incest taboo and of organized society, but she enriches the myth also with a mother figure, belonging to the initial period before the development of language (both historically and in the development of each human individual).[42] Kristeva works here with Freud's general idea that human reactions to defilement must be seen in the context of how human identity as a rational being is established. It is a process in which humans are required to distance themselves from nature, the nature for which dirt stands as the main symbol. However, Kristeva's general attitude seems somewhat different from Freud's. Unlike Freud, she suggests not only that our experiences of dread, disgust and abjection threaten our existential confidence in a meaningful reality. She also thinks they constitute an opening towards a valuable if unutterable truth.

Kristeva is doubtlessly familiar with Sartre's *Nausea*, but the crucial elements of her theory at this juncture bear the fingerprints of Bataille rather than Sartre. In unmistakable references to Bataille's Heterology, Kristeva speaks of 'abjections' which she sees as originating in the infantile need to establish an identity separate from the mother. The personal development of the child, its process of individuation – whereby it learns to think of itself as a unique being, a subject facing an external world of objects – must start with a basic demarcation. The child must cut itself off from the mother and constitute itself as a body of its own. Ritual cleanliness, as reinforcement and reaffirmation of bodily integrity, is an expression of the refusal to be once more swallowed up by the mother – the all-embracing Mother which is also Nature.[43]

Kristeva roots her interpretation of filth in an idea of the relationship between the ego and the non-ego or the alien. *Threat towards bodily integrity* becomes the paradigm case, and dirt is presented as a borderline phenomenon: something sticky that challenges the purity and independent existence of the human body.[44] At this juncture, Kristeva makes skilful use of the French word *propre*, translated as 'clean', 'proper' and 'own'. In graphic images of decay, nausea and dread, she describes how in my reactions to waste matter, 'I give birth to myself amid the violence of sobs, of vomit.'[45] The birth of the subject and its demarcation against the Mother is constantly re-enacted in my reactions. My ability to establish myself as an individual is the necessary condition of meaningful thinking, logic and language, and abjection is my way of guarding the possibility of meaning. In this context, the body of the mother represents an archaic force, on the near side of separation, unconscious, tempting us to the point of losing our differences, our speech, our life; to the point of aphasia, decay, opprobrium, and death.[46]

When abjection is assigned a fundamental role in culture, theoretical conditions are also created for unmasking our support for hygiene and the *propre*, usually understood as a sound and responsible attitude towards one's physical environment, as something grounded in the subject's primitive need to guard itself against threats of dissolution. Dirt, refuse, cadavers and excrements *are made* filthy because they are declared non-objects of desire.

Abjection works both at the level of individuals and at the level of societies, which use it to consolidate social boundaries. In a reading inspired by Douglas and Freud, Kristeva subjects Mosaic Law to psychoanalytical reinterpretation. Its rules of ritual purity are, as with Freud, derived from the incest taboo – in the last analysis, the attempt to control access to the Mother.[47] Kristeva relies here on extended chains of associations, in one sense surprising and in another sense utterly predictable for those who know the theoretical tradition.[48] For the present purposes we should, however, not try to judge Kristeva's theory of abjection by its historical plausibility but by its role in *contemporary* debate.

If the paradigm of abjection is a myth, then it should be assessed according to the inspiratory powers that it has. Does it make things clearer; is it any good for the social causes towards which it has been harnessed? Sociologist Imogen Tyler notes that Kristeva's book was widely hailed among English-speaking scholars and activists as a resource for feminism.[49] However, she objects, women are only present in it in the form of the abject maternal body, while the thinking subject is described in *opposition* to the Mother. Kristeva's book completely ignores the female experience of *being* a mother: 'Indeed the fundamental premise of the Kristevan abject is that there is and can be no maternal subject' – and in this way, *Powers of Horror* risks reproducing rather than challenging the disgust towards female reproduction.[50] Kristeva speaks of the subject's dread of the other, but she does not inquire into the subjectivity of those on whose lot it falls to be such 'others'.

Tyler points out that the same problem is present in Kristeva's contribution to a second debate in which she is frequently cited, namely one addressing national identity, racism and xenophobia. In work published after *Powers of Horror*, Kristeva takes up these themes, but also here Tyler presents a very damaging critique.[51] According to Kristeva, xenophobia is one more expression of the primal rejection of the mother. The foreigner is a substitute for the abject maternal, which symbolically poses a threat to the political body of the nation state. Kristeva's cure is psychoanalysis and her final aim is to develop a politics of 'cosmopolitan hospitality' towards strangers. However, in a strange *volte-face* after these promising beginnings, Kristeva identifies cosmopolitanism with the officially universalistic 'good' nationalism of the French Republic[52] – while minority groups, especially Muslim women with scarves, stand for the rejection of cosmopolitan values.[53] Thus, starting off from a purported critique of xenophobia, she ends up denouncing the usual suspects as abject and alien elements inside the pure body of the republic.

The xenophobe says, 'It is *us* against *them*. After years and years of humanitarian bombing those ingrates are still not shaping up. All Arabs should go to Arabia, Jews to Judea and Indians to Indiana.' One hardly needs to be a celebrated literary theorist to see how daft *that* is. The question is how to see xenophobia in context. Tyler remarks that a central problem of Kristeva's theory is precisely its aspiration to universality: psychoanalysis is supposed to be valid regardless of time and place and hence the rejection of strangers must lie in human nature. Tyler calls instead for informative accounts of social exclusion that pay heed to the specific historical situation of Europe, especially including its colonial past and the present dismantling of the welfare state.

The strength, or weakness if you will, of myths – the abjection paradigm not excluded – lies precisely in their universality, the possibility of applying them on more or less everything. Universal applicability, however, makes very vague concepts. 'Heterogeneity' in Bataille's and Kristeva's hands is 'abject' and marked by disgust and dread, but in the end this strikes me as a rather bad description of our most usual attitudes towards soiling and refuse (and towards foreigners and mothers) – ever so many supporting literary examples notwithstanding. It seems to me that dirt and waste matter are most of the time not *simply* rejected but they have quite definite places in the cultural system. For instance, we discuss them and work with them; we do not just shy away from 'abject matter' in total incomprehension. In one sense, abject theory comes up against the old Platonic problem of identifying the Form of something that is supposed to be Form-less. If dirt is just *rejected*, how can Bataille and Kristeva ever write about it?

Immanuel Kant, Émile Durkheim and the categories of thought

What of the great project, the naturalization of the categories? Was it finally demonstrated that the possibility of thought depends on socially instituted patterns of order and exclusion?

Durkheim conceived of his theory as a rejection of Kant's, but at at least one level Kant might have agreed as a matter of course that our ways of thinking are influenced by culture and biology.[54] It is only that *that* was not a theme for his *Critique* and above all it was not the fish he had to fry. His question was not how thinking is influenced but what thinking *is*. Durkheim believed that space, time and the categories constrict thinking; Kant believed they make thinking possible, or perhaps, that they *are* our thinking.

Durkheim stressed the importance, for social cohesion, that everyone in society should 'have the same conception of time, space, cause, number, etc.'[55] The important phrase here is '*conception* of . . .'

In relation to temporality, it would imply members of society sharing agreed ways of dividing time into measurable units for the sake of coordinated action. Kant's point was much more fundamental, for he argued that temporality as such is an organizing principle of our experience, regardless of culturally specific ways of measuring time. In a society, different ways of conceptualizing time may be imaginable, but in order for the individual to understand temporal classifications as 'conceptions of *time*' temporality must be assumed from the start. Durkheim failed to see the separateness of these two issues and the fundamental point that, as Steven Lukes points out, 'we cannot postulate a hypothetical situation in which individuals do not in general think by means of space, time, class, person, cause and according to the rules of logic, since this is what thinking is.'[56] Another way to formulate the Kantian position is to say that for Kant, *necessity* is one of the categories, and therefore it will not be meaningful to ask whether the categories themselves are necessary – by pain of ending up with nonsense questions like, 'Why is necessity necessary?' or 'Why is logic logical?' None of this is to claim that Kant is untouchable. But the naturalization of the categories and the forms of intuition is not a coherent project if presented as a response to Kant.

One might suggest that the merits of the myth of abjection should be assessed, not with regard to theoretical coherence but in terms of its capacity to inspire social criticism and emancipatory action. A question here is to what extent those potentialities are compromised by the paradigm's uncleared-up background in racist and patriarchal discourses of the early twentieth century. Does the paradigm of abjection disentangle those discourses or does it reproduce them? Socially vulnerable groups like immigrants and pregnant mothers might not appreciate being singled out as 'abject'. And citizens of the global South will hardly be jumping up and down in joy at being compared with children and neurotics.

SEVEN

The Civilizing Process

Norbert Elias and the civilizing process

Are we less dirty now than we were a hundred, three hundred, a thousand years ago? If so, is it because we now have warm water taps in the house and we didn't then? Or is there generally less tolerance towards dirt in modern society? If that is true, what does that say about our culture as a whole?

The answers will in part depend on who 'we' are supposed to be, where, and what time of the day and the week. A European tenant farmer three hundred years ago, in the middle of a workday, would smell more strongly of sweat than, say, an accountant would do today, if only because of the general difference that still exists between outdoor and indoor jobs. In precisely the same way, we would expect different average levels of personal hygiene from those with access to bathrooms and showers and those (for instance, in traditional peasant societies) who must make do with a bucket of water in the shared kitchen-cum-living area. General changes in economy, housing and living standards in the industrialized parts of the world point to the conclusion that 'we' on the whole, at least for most hours of the day, are cleaner than the majority were three hundred years ago – however, allowing for variation according to geography and social class.[1] It stands to reason that general tolerance towards soiling and bad hygiene in Western societies was previously higher than today *on average*, because one must presume that recognized standards bear some reasonable relation to what is agreed to be realistic; but none of this is yet to give any verdict about whether the *ideal* itself has changed. In other words: granted that people in the past sometimes were forced to tolerate more dirt than we do today, is there any reason to think that they still did not perceive filth precisely as filth and stench precisely as stench?

In response to this question, several scholars today would argue that modern restrictive attitudes towards dirt are a recent development, and they would refer to *Norbert Elias* and his work *The Civilizing Process* for confirmation.[2] In two bulky volumes, Elias described the development of Western civilization, *the birth of the modern individual*, as a process of increasing self-discipline, a central part of which consisted in raised standards of personal hygiene. With modernization, we are told, the principal means for socially controlling individuals switched from *external* to *internal* pressure.[3] According to Elias, the main method for instilling this new form of self-discipline in early modern men and women was by evoking intensified feelings of shame and disgust. Starting approximately at the time of the Reformation, people were not only brought to believe that natural functions of the human body – metabolism, sexuality, illness and death – had to be concealed, had to be kept exclusively for the individuals concerned;[4] but moreover, a private sphere was created, the boundaries of which would shield the individual against physical intimacy.[5]

If then Elias accounts for the modern individual's (allegedly) lowered tolerance of dirt above all in terms of an instinctive but socially inculcated wish to keep the surrounding world at bay, then the opposite was apparently true of the people of the Middle Ages. According to Lorentz Lyttkens, who elaborates on Elias, medieval man was 'not an isolated being' but his characteristic feature consisted in '"admixture" with other men, with created things, with demons, with beasts tame and wild in the environment'.[6] Consequently 'it was often unclear where a person would end and the environment would start.'[7] This was clearly visible at the dining table, where eating with one's fingers was natural because 'no sharp boundaries were drawn between meal and man'.[8] In this sense, the medievals were like children and their world view was undifferentiated and magical.[9] The affinity with Freud's views is unmistakable. Just as the maturation of the human individual is a replay of the development of the entire species, the history of modern Western civilization involves increase of the kind of self-discipline that marks the adult from the child.[10]

This view of the civilizing process is one version of the theories of modernity that have been around for about as long as there has been modernity to devise theories about. David Hume believed in the gradual softening and refinement of manners. Rousseau also believed that such development had taken place, only adding that it was a form of corruption brought about by twisted social conditions. One more important precursor to Elias is his fellow sociologist Max Weber and his theory of the successive rationalization of Western society under capitalism. Interesting specific features about Elias were his attention to seemingly banal details of everyday life as markers of general changes in mentality, his ability to connect those details to changes of social structure, and his incorporation of the (originally Freudian) concept of the unconscious. In these respects, he arrived independently and somewhat ahead of time at a research approach reminiscent of the French *Annales* School.[11]

Elias published his book in 1939, but its main impact on scholarship came only as a new edition was published in 1969 and translated from the original German to several languages in the late 1970s and early '80s. The idea of a civilizing and rationalizing process became standard fare in literature on the history of manners – and this to the extent that, according to one critic, Elias is routinely cited in introductory sections also of mainly unconnected work simply for greater rhetorical dignity, just as it was once *de rigueur* to quote classical poets or founding fathers of 'scientific Marxism'.[12]

The heritage industry has happily embraced the idea of a civilizing process, but exclusively out of interest in the contrasting Dark Ages that it must imply. It may not be easy to re-enact a vanished life form, but there is money to be made especially from the carnival aspects of Ye Olde Forme of life. The theory of the civilizing process is alive and well in my home town, just a stone's throw away from my bedroom window. Whatever you might think, the functionaries of the annual Medieval Fayre are neither touched in the head nor drunk; they are just acting out the Grand Narrative of Western Civilization. As the brochure tells us, 'The Medievals lived in the here and now' – 'When there was feasting and frolicking, it was for real' – 'In the Middle Ages anything might happen. The experience is difficult to describe'.[13]

The brochure might easily cite Elias for learned support, for the medievals lived, according to him, in a world that 'oscillates between extremes'.[14] Men abandoned themselves to wild pleasures, their desire for women, their hate, their fears;[15] in comparison with modern men they were 'incomparably more ready and accustomed to leap with undiminishing intensity from one extreme to the other, and slight impressions, uncontrollable associations [were] often enough to induce these immense fluctuations'.[16]

It is part of this general picture that people in the Middle Ages and up to the early modern period had a *natural and uncompli-cated* relation to their own filth and stench, not associating the offices of nature with any sense of shame whatever – which explains why there were, according to Elias, no spaces specifically set apart for that purpose. The medievals could quite simply relieve them-selves on the street, in the middle of a conversation or during a meal. Good examples supposedly to this effect are included in the gen-erally very readable collection of essays by the Swedish historian Peter Englund, devoting a chapter to 'Stench and Filth'.[17] Englund reproduces a story about Louis XIV of France who was 'not ashamed to empty his bowels, sitting on the night-stool, with the royal house-hold crowding in on him like a herd of carefully drilled French poodles', as well as a description of Anne Boleyn who 'did not leave the table when she needed to shit during her coronation banquet, but simply let herself be shielded by a linen sheet'.[18]

According to Elias, a definitive transformation in the European mindset occurred in the seventeenth and eighteenth centuries, involving a transformation of the ideal from *courtoisie* to *civilité*. His most important source material consists of guidebooks of polite behaviour, which indicate a gradual rise of the standards of propriety. It was made obligatory to blow one's nose in a handkerchief and not in a hand or a sleeve. It was now forbidden to eat with one's fingers and to urinate and break wind in the presence of others. Above all people were made to feel that the natural functions of the human body were shameful and had to be discharged without anyone noticing. The starting point of this gradual change was court society, from where polite manners spread 'downwards' and outwards like rings on water. Their absolute centre lay in Versailles – that is, in France, the kingdom where tendencies towards administrative centralization flourished earlier than elsewhere in Europe. In feudal society there had been 'no central power strong enough to compel people to restraint'.[19] Now with increased division of labour in society at large, chains of social interdependence became steadily longer, connecting every part of society with every other. The rise of a centralized state, with the monopoly of legitimate use of force, was a decisive factor, because aristocracy, once a relatively independent warrior class with access to private fortresses, was reduced to a stratum of loyal courtiers and administrators. The personal career of a nobleman no longer depended on his military prowess, but on cutting a fine figure at court.

Those destined for success had to learn self-discipline from early on. A strong control of impulses was required, something that still is the case in modern society; only today it has become a pressure that we hardly notice because it is such an obvious part of normal education.[20] There is, however, a price to pay. We have been encumbered with 'a specific "super-ego", which endeavours to control, transform or suppress [our] affects in keeping with the social structure', giving rise to damaging psychological conflicts inside each individual.[21] Quoting Elias once more:

But the drives, the passionate affects, that can no longer directly manifest themselves in the relationships *between* people, often struggle no less violently *within* the individual against this supervising part of himself. And this semi-automatic struggle of the person with himself does not always find a happy resolution . . . The vertical oscillations, if we may so describe them, the leaps from fear to joy, pleasure to remorse are reduced, while the horizontal fissure running right through the whole person, the tension between 'super-ego' and 'unconscious' – the wishes and desires that cannot be remembered – increases.[22]

Elias apparently shares Freud's misgivings about civilization and its discontents, but unlike Freud he describes the dynamic of ego and superego as a specific feature of a particular historical period, that of European modernity, owing its existence to the modern need for intensified self-control.

The history of shit in the modern period

The general narrative, where the modern era is characterized by the constant increase of discipline, has been embraced by others independently of Elias. Thus for Michel Foucault, European cultural development from the sixteenth century onwards (the same period that Elias was interested in) started with the tightening of mechanisms of repression and control, later however giving way to self-surveillance, whereby every individual is now his or her own thought police.

The idea of discipline as the key to modern subjectivity is made to bear directly on the origins of modern hygiene in Dominique Laporte's *Histoire de la merde (prologue)*, translated as *History of Shit*.[23] Published 1978, the book mainly focuses on the same 'classical epoch' of *c.* 1500–1800 that Foucault covered in his genealogies of the asylum, the prison and sexuality in the 1960s and '70s. The nominal theme of *Histoire de la merde* is the management of waste in (mostly French) cities, but Laporte paints a much broader picture where society as a whole undergoes systematic streamlining and organizing efforts. The book itself originally came about as a kind of by-product – or, as his posthumous editor suggests, 'recycled waste' – of Laporte's research on the history of the French language.[24] Starting in the sixteenth century, French scholars and administrators made systematic efforts to create a standardized idiom to serve the needs of the centralized French state. Just as the language of the king and his realm were to be cleansed of excesses and foreign elements, so would the public spaces of the king's capital.

> One can speak of a politics of waste in the sixteenth century, if it is understood in terms of a slow process of repression – one that only achieves its goal in the golden age of capitalism and is hastened by socialism's reduction of man to his needs.[25]

There is *merde* both in the city and in language, and for this reason 'civilization's ambivalence toward shit' still shows itself in both domains; 'on the one hand, by a will to wash those places where garbage collects (i.e., in city and speech) and, on the other, by a belief in the purifying value of waste – so long as it is human'.[26] The crux of the matter is that *merde*, including dirt and waste in the broadest sense possible, was already in the early modern age *not* perceived simply as a practical problem of hygiene, for 'hygiene's true drive is located far from its purported aim'.[27] The real aim of the purifying efforts, by means of a more efficient control of the private lives of citizens, lay in the very fact of *control as such*. The introduction of secluded outhouses and privies separated from the bedroom in the sixteenth century paved the way for the forms of affect control characteristic of the bourgeois family and bourgeois public space in nineteenth-century capitalism.

The (Freudian) 'symbolic equation of money and shit' runs through Laporte's book as a red thread.[28] There were profits to be made when public management of waste transformed 'impure' shit into 'pure' fertilizer. Quite similarly, the state provided methods by which the individual capitalist could have his dirty money laundered and thus gain entry to the social elite in accordance with 'Vespasian's axiom', *pecunia non olet* – 'money has no smell'.[29]

On the whole, then, the message from scholarly debates appears to be this: feelings of shame for one's body functions are neither biologically given nor a universal feature of human societies, but rather they were once forced down the throats of early modern men and women. The birth of modern subjectivity was the result of those disciplinary efforts.

What do the documents say?

On closer inspection, however, the grand narrative does not quite square with evidence. Empirical research on the development of West European personal hygiene suggests a U-shaped curve rather than linear ascent. The sixteenth and seventeenth centuries saw deterioration, gradually to be reversed towards the end of the eighteenth century.[30] Two main reasons account for the lowering of hygienic standards in the early modern age: the increase of urban density and, partly as a consequence of that trend, the diminished use of water between 1550 and 1750. Both the quality and availability of water generally suffered because of inadequate infrastructures in the rapidly growing and industrializing cities.[31] The empirical material has limitations, however. The lives of ordinary people are generally not well documented and, especially when it comes to details about cleanliness, there is some risk of tendentious descriptions.

The influence from ideology is conspicuous when we compare two descriptions of supposedly pre-modern or less than fully modern hygiene, both from 1938. The Swedish journalist

Ludvig Nordström contributed to the debate of his time on hygienic reforms with a report that is still widely cited. As indicated by the title *Lort-Sverige* (Filth Sweden), Nordström's report condemned traditional rural dwellings as unhealthy, filthy and smelly.[32] That same year, ethnologist Kustaa Vilkuna published a study of peasant milieus in southwest Finland, documenting mainly homesteads of small but independent farmers. The two regions are geographically close and the folk culture is for a large part indistinguishable. Quite in contrast to Nordström, however, Vilkuna stressed the cleanliness of the homes that he in some cases had personally visited for documentation.[33] Clearly the two authors were following different agendas. Nordström wanted to contribute to debates on social reform while Vilkuna may have been influenced by traditional ethnographic commitments to local patriotism and nation-building.

We may expect the perils of ideology to grow even further with the increase of historical distance to whatever is described. Consider the entrenched idea of the medieval city as steeped in filth and stench. Modern writers love to dwell on descriptions that supposedly prove exactly that; however, art historian Johann Konrad Eberlein states that the documentation for this conception hardly goes beyond the level of sources like city guides.[34] According to Hans Peter Duerr, before the rapid urban growth of the modern era, the smell in cities and towns was probably not more disturbing than it would be in an ordinary farmhouse.[35] This is reasonable concerning the fact that the amount of human faeces produced in a medieval or early modern city was dwarfed by animal dung – a hundred cows or two hundred horses produce roughly the same amount of manure as a town of four to five thousand inhabitants – thus the smell of human excrement was hardly dominant.[36] In addition, outhouses were routinely placed next to the dung-heap so that human and animal droppings were naturally mixed. What, on the other hand, was missing in the medieval urban environment was motor traffic constantly whipping up dust from the streets.[37]

If we try to get an idea of the hygiene standards of years past we need the critical methods of historical research. We must think of the context of the damning descriptions; by *whom* they were produced, under what circumstances, and for whom. If a certain milieu is described as filthy, strictly speaking we only know that the author believed it was, or for some reason wanted others to believe it was, or wanted others to believe that *he* thus believed. Elias does not pause to reflect on this, which is why there is a certain unwitting irony in his use of sources. For example, he cites from *Colloquia familiaria* by Erasmus of Rotterdam. In one of the fictive dialogues included in Erasmus' book, the sad state of German inns is contrasted with the clean, inexpensive and friendly service available in Lyons, France. Elias seizes on this polemic against German conditions, taking it to be a faithful description of general housing standards for travellers at the time (Erasmus, he tells us, is 'forced by the subject itself to adhere closely to social reality', which 'he finds present in social life itself').[38] As historian Gerd Schwerhoff points out, if Elias had chosen instead to focus on Erasmus' description of Lyonnais inns included in the same dialogue, he could easily have presented the sixteenth century in a very 'modern' light.[39] Moreover, the dialogue itself goes to show that Erasmus was *not* indifferent to hygiene and that he expected his readers to share his sentiments. Insofar as early observers were genuinely shocked by low levels of cleanliness, by the same token we learn that their general expectations were higher. None of this indicates that early modern Europeans were not troubled by bad hygienic standards.[40]

A similar point applies to the allegedly impulsive and quarrelsome personalities of medieval and early modern men and women.[41] For instance, seventeenth-century court records attest to violent conflicts about symbolic status such as seating in church, with one burgher refusing to give up his pew to another. How could they get worked up about such trifles? Here too we must think of the context where such events were *recorded*. Apparently these incidents became court cases exactly because impolite and quarrelsome behaviour was *not* the norm – and therefore these conflicts were not about trifles. Social status was not inessential for a burgher who wished to maintain his good name. That went as far as to the assignment of seats in churches, while modern people might from the perspective of the past be accused of carelessness, since we just do not seem to think of where we seat ourselves.

Critical reflection on the use of sources is on the whole absent in *The Civilizing Process*, which has given professional historians reason for criticism. However, the most vocal criticism in the debate comes from ethnologist Hans Peter Duerr and his book *Der Mythos vom Zivilisationsprozess* (The Myth of the Civilizing Process). In that voluminous work, Duerr makes wide use of the kind of material that Elias has cited, sometimes including the very same sources, but his conclusions are quite the opposite. He massively disconfirms the thesis that it was only with the onset of modernity that human body functions began to be perceived as embarrassing. Such embarrassment is, for instance, strongly developed among so called primitive or pre-modern peoples.[42] In fact Duerr believes it is a universal human trait; 'there is a lot to say for the truth of the biblical myth that shame for exposing the genital area is not historically contingent but rather belongs to human *essence*.'[43] While the claim to universality might be too simplified,[44] Duerr has certainly demonstrated that the association of human body functions and nakedness with shame is not just a recent European invention and that it does not owe its existence to the rise of the centralized state.

One example is the evacuation of the bowels, which, *pace* Elias, would have been far from a normal thing to do in the presence of others during the European Middle Ages.[45] Not only were there secluded places of ease, but in speech they were designated with various euphemisms such as 'privie', 'wardrobe', 'necessary house' or quite simply the place '*qui n'est pas honneste a nommer*' (which it is not decent to name).[46] During the Renaissance and up to the eighteenth century, the elite favoured the portable night-stool, which could be comfortably used in heated rooms and then emptied by servants, but the sense of shame came into play again: a whole range of euphemisms was invented for this piece of furniture, and it was disguised, for instance, as a trunk or as a pile of books so as not to embarrass visitors.[47] In his famous guidebook of manners for children, *De civilitate* (1530), Erasmus advises the reader always to excuse himself in advance if he has to mention things that might disgust the listener, such as vomiting, the outhouse or faeces.[48] Duerr concludes: 'We see in other words that Norbert Elias, to say the least, overstates his case when he writes that people in the time of Erasmus could still talk quite naturally about things that are today concealed behind a wall of silence.'[49]

What, then, Duerr asks, about the frequently quoted descriptions of how highly-placed French aristocrats would receive guests while sitting on the night-stool? Duerr argues that this form of socializing, known in English as 'the French courtesy', was not an archaic remnant of medieval manners, but a specifically French phenomenon, developed in the seventeenth and early eighteenth centuries as a way of showing off one's superiority and indicating that the guest was not particularly honoured.[50] To cite cases of this kind as examples of a general freedom of manners will be misleading, at least if one fails to mention that those at the receiving end perceived such freedom as both remarkable and insulting.[51] Thus if Anne Boleyn could permit herself to sit on the chamber-pot during her coronation banquet – unseen, behind a curtain – the message was not that other members of the party could have taken (or even wanted) such liberties.

These social or semi-public events are one thing; it is another thing that there really was no such thing as private life for the French king, for he constantly had a page or servant on his side. When Christian VII of Denmark during his visit of 1768 asked for a private interview with Louis XV, he was politely but firmly refused for two reasons: the king was not alone for a single minute of his life, 'not even in the privy' (*garderobe*), and secondly, the king could not turn out persons who, in virtue of their rank and privileges, had the right to be present in his rooms.[52] This description indicates that, while the king did not enjoy privacy of any kind, this was not due to any generally *careless* attitude about forms of socializing. It indicates, on the contrary, a formal or ceremonial setting with little room for the kind of impulsive behaviour that, for instance, Elias would associate with medieval times and early modernity.

EIGHT

Ambiguities of Self-discipline and the Campaign for Civilization

The idea of self-discipline

The onset of modernity from the Renaissance onwards is typically represented as involving the increase of self-discipline in everyday life. Hans Peter Duerr, however, makes in his book some observations that demonstrate the ambiguity of this concept. He claims that public urination was unacceptable in the Middle Ages, just as it is in our own time and generally has been in human culture,[1] even though it is in practice often overlooked, at least in the male case. The implicit rule in those cases is for passers-by to behave as if they had not seen anything.[2] Which, however, gives a peculiar twist to the question of self-discipline – namely: who is now the undisciplined one? The one who urinates or the one who looks on? Devoting a chapter of his book to 'the indiscreet gaze', Duerr argues that lack of self-restraint is not necessarily shown by those who show themselves (partly) naked but by those (for instance, European anthropologists) who cannot keep their eyes off them.[3] He notes on the subject of traditional Japanese bathing customs:

> The fact of both sexes bathing naked together by no means indicates – unlike what, for instance, Elias believes – that the limits of shame are less strongly felt in this case than when the bathers are dressed. On the contrary, the mixed bath seems to have required a higher degree of 'drive abstention', because one had, on the one hand, perpetually to be on one's guard so as to keep one's eyes from wandering

and yet on the other hand, especially in the case of women, to be constantly aware that others would be seeing or even looking at the most intimate parts of one's body. The result was an atmosphere of control rather than the one of ease that Western observers, one after another, thought they could sense.[4]

A similar point is made about mixed bathing in the Finnish sauna.[5] Quite early on, travellers from central Europe to northern Finland were thrilled by the idea of men, women and children sitting together stark naked, presenting it to their home market as an exotic case of pre-modern 'natural' attitudes towards the body.[6] On the other hand, reformers in Finland condemned the joint bath as shameless and barbarian.[7] In any case, it was a more interesting story to take home than the also frequent practice of separate bathing for men and women.[8] The Italian traveller Giuseppe Acerbi reported in 1802 that men and women would sit in the bath side by side, 'without . . . being in the least influenced by any emotions of attachment'. He then added an important detail:

> If, however, a stranger open the door, and come on the bathers by surprise, the women are not a little startled at his appearance; for, besides his person, he introduces along with him, by opening the door, a great quantity of light, which discovers at once to the view their situation, as well as forms . . . I often amused myself with surprising the bathers in this manner.[9]

Who are the ones giving free rein to their impulses in this story – the 'pre-modern' bathers or Cavaliere Acerbi amusing himself?

In any case, a general point should be made. The difference between the reactions of Acerbi and the bathers has an obvious parallel in the discrepancies between Elias and Duerr. Culturally imposed discipline may affirm itself in opposite ways: the offending element may either be put literally out of sight (for example, behind a partition wall) or it may be made 'invisible' by looking away from it or ignoring it.

This argument gives us a new way of interpreting Anne Boleyn's predicament at her coronation banquet. The dinner was a ceremonial occasion with the royal couple at its absolute centre, sitting on thrones at a table and facing hundreds of guests as well as servants and onlookers. Had the Queen now excused herself, leaving the room, she would have interrupted or even caused the cessation of the festive occasion, thus drawing explicit attention to the unmentionable 'private matter'.

The general idea that the introduction of modernity coincides with the increase of self-discipline and the increasing obsession with hygiene has the appearance of a *historical* thesis.[10] Modernization is seen as a process whereby dirt is made taboo and banished from society, as habitual disgust of dirt is being inculcated by means of socially imposed discipline. However, for the thesis to be properly historical, specific details should be presented of the distribution, respectively, of repressive and permissive attitudes in the milieus at issue. Statements concerning 'pre-modern' as opposed to 'modern Bourgeois' or 'Victorian' cultures suffer from the frequent failure to specify the milieus and situations to which they are meant to be applicable. As a reviewer of Frykman's work on the development of cleanliness in Sweden has remarked, we are left in the dark as to the time period, social class and indeed home country of the 'Victorian'; he 'sometimes hails from the 1950s and sometimes he is a mad German doctor of old' – but is '*never a clearly defined group of people with a specific economic and social standing*'.[11] We meet with the same kind of vagueness if we try to pin down the contrasting 'pre-modern' individual. The 'premodern' sometimes inhabits a medieval town, sometimes the French court in the eighteenth century and sometimes a farm in southern Sweden in the 1930s.

Water-based and order-based cleanliness

One factor, more than anything else, is probably responsible for confusion about 'pre-modern' attitudes to dirt. Most studies by anthropologists and cultural historians concern the lives of people who – unlike *them* but not unlike the present majority of living human beings – have only limited access to clean water. Those of us who live in the industrialized West typically enjoy forms of hygiene based on the use of water, while hygiene in other milieus is to a large extent based on *keeping order*.[12] To cite an example that might be familiar to readers who have spent time camping or in primitive summer homes: instead of washing up after breakfast, teacups, knives and forks may be left in place for everyone to find their own for later use. The general principle of hygiene based on order is aimed at minimizing the points of contact between clean and dirty items.

European languages have retained some reminiscences of order-based hygiene. The Swedish word for *right* (as opposed to left), *höger*, conserves the memory of Indo-European practices where cleanliness was apparently based on the interplay of two contrasts, juxtaposing the conceptual pair 'right/left' with 'higher/lower' (cf. *högre*, 'higher'). The physical boundary between high and low was drawn at the waist. Unclean items of the 'lower' sphere were only to be touched with the left hand, leaving the right hand free for 'higher' pursuits. Thus the right hand was 'right' also in the sense of being proper for such tasks, and this hierarchical relation is reproduced in several languages.[13]

In North Europe, the culture of the Roma ('gypsies') has preserved a comprehensive form of hygiene based on order up to the present times. Among the Finnish Roma cleanliness implied that kitchen utensils, should they for some reason touch the floor, could no longer be used for cooking even after careful cleaning.[14] Men's and women's clothes, underwear and over-clothing, must be washed and hung separately as well as kept separate;[15] people of symbolically inferior position (women, young men) were not supposed to place themselves physically above people of higher position (for example, upstairs in a house) lest they symbolically contaminate those underneath.[16] As to menstruation, the Finnish Roma, unlike most Roma communities, had no specific pollution taboos – according to sociologist Martti Grönfors, simply because the culture as a whole was based on 'an extreme denial of sexuality', which is why it was not possible even to formulate regulations about the topic.[17]

It is obvious from these descriptions that the relevant principles of order are not only about cleanliness in the restricted sense, but that they connect with a general pattern of propriety and respect in the best spirit of Mary Douglas. Hygiene based on order works well in conditions of scarcity, but it is naturally not a very flexible system, which is why it is less functional in societies that involve division of labour, requiring frequent contacts between interacting social groups. Order-based hygiene naturally leads to situations where entire professional categories become untouchable if they, for work reasons, cannot avoid contact with uncleanliness. Thus Aljosha Taikon, of the Swedish Roma, tells us in his autobiography, *Aljosha: Son of the Gypsy Chief*, that he could no longer be invited for coffee after he had started working for the Swedish National Health Service. He would wear a white coat and gloves for work and wash his hands hundreds of times every day, but he would not be allowed to touch the china of other Roma families.[18]

Quite probably our general assessments of hygienic standards in cultures other than the current Western mainstream are shaped by the fact that we tend to expect solutions based on water rather than order. For instance, Englund has described the cleanliness of seventeenth-century European aristocracy as a form of early modern 'cheat hygiene', implying that this social stratum still harboured a completely natural and unconstrained attitude (unlike *ours*) towards body waste and stench:

Three methods were in use . . . The first consisted in wiping. Instead of dabbling in water, people would wipe off the filth with dry cloths and moist towels (bran and different types of powder were employed for washing the hair, for not even this part of the body should be wetted without good reason. Often the method was to rub in the substance before going to bed and then to comb it off in the morning.) The second means was the perfumed powder . . . The fine scent would cover up for minor hygienic blemishes . . . The third and most important method consisted in the use of linen. The secret of the dry cleanliness was that linen was worn next to the body and these garments were changed frequently.[19]

On closer inspection, however, nothing in this description of water-free hygiene indicates that the early modern aristocrat did not perceive dirt and smell as disturbing. There was only a minimal use of water, but the hair was washed with powder. Why was water avoided? Well, water 'was seen as a carrier of contagion',[20] not an unrealistic consideration in the circumstances. Englund is, however, looking at his sources through the same 'civilizing' spectacles as Elias. Social development is described as a streamlining process where emotional impulses, including sexuality, sobbing, laughing, sloth and even courage, are gradually brought under control.

This constant theme of Englund's collection of essays corresponds to a similar trend in the descriptions offered by Jonas Frykman. Frykman operates with the opposing poles of bourgeois discipline and rural freedom of constraint. Describing the hygienic practices in a household of Swedish agricultural workers around 1910, he works himself up about the 'specific reservoirs of filth' contained in the kitchen-cum-living room: the slop-pail, the spittoon, the snot-rag, the chamber-pot placed under the bedstead.[21] Considering Frykman's troubles with these items, we might of course ask what, for him, would have been the preferable way to dispose of filth in a household that lacks running water, tissues and drains to flush turds away to . . . some place or other of which we mostly have no idea.

The conflict between old and new methods of cleanliness was sometimes also expressed with humour. This is how Edward 'Edo' Nordman, when he later worked as keeper at the outdoor museum of Sagalund in Kimito, Finland, would describe the cottage where he was born and bred along with seven siblings – and 'we all lived there 'til we were dead'. The custom was for all members of the household to eat with their own wooden spoons which they would then lick or wipe clean and place on a shelf.

> He [Nordman] was also of the opinion that the cause of all modern diseases lay in the excess of cleanliness and he had a theory of his own about how tuberculosis came to spread in the region: 'Year 1882 was when consumption came here, before that we'd all eat with the same spoon from the same pot and the germs would gobble each other up.'[22]

Instead of linear progress, it is more realistic to speak of competing cleanliness cultures, old and new, in rural areas entering modernity. For instance, well into the twentieth century, Finnish country folk resisted the urban use of handkerchiefs. The handkerchief was surely appreciated as a decorative status symbol, for instance to be used by women for pointedly wiping tears during a church service; but to employ it for its original purpose and then to fold it into one's pocket with the snot and all would have been simply uncouth.[23] This is hardly an indication that these 'premodern' or less than fully modern peasants were indifferent to body waste.

This not-fully-modern conception of cleanliness was intimately connected with what we today would think of as 'quite another thing'; for instance, to be properly groomed was part of what it meant to show respect to the elderly. We are still not completely foreign to these associations, even if they are largely lost on us if we just think of cleanliness as personal hygiene. On the other hand, the contrast between water-based hygiene and hygiene based on order is not absolute, for both serve the goal of creating an agreeable and healthy human environment. Moreover, when we clean with water we also must follow our routines in a certain order. Washing up after a meal, we take the glasses first and the pots and pans in the end; washing the floor, we start by the window and work our way towards the door.

On the whole there is a certain cultural myopia involved in the idea that 'pre-moderns' did not care about cleanliness but only about order. A visiting 'pre-modern' observer would commit a similar, although opposite, mistake if they were to conclude that 'moderns' just care about splashing in water and not about cleanliness.

Varieties of refinement

The difficulty of recognizing forms of cleanliness different from one's own is illustrative of the kind of home blindness we must always try to avoid in our descriptions of long-term cultural change. In the development of humanity, it is not only the quantity of what is done that has undergone changes, but its quality; we need to see that at some point or other the appropriate measuring rods are no longer the same as before. Or, to be more precise: with the increase of the historical span the span of ambiguity about interpretations also increases. It becomes impossible for us positively to identify any cultural change as *simply* quantitative. Norbert Elias of course in some sense emphasizes the 'otherness' of the pre-moderns, and thus the qualitative difference between them and us, when he insists that the people whose life he describes did not feel the same need to restrain their emotional impulses as we do. But it appears to me that he makes the pre-moderns *more* foreign than one need to, precisely because he does not recognize the differences between modern and earlier perceptions of what *counts as* restraint or lack thereof.

Cultural development has no doubt given rise to new forms of constraint and mutual respect, but it has also involved the disappearance of earlier forms. Narratives that only trace the gradual emergence of self-discipline as we today know it are constitutionally blind to its other forms – which is of course connected to the fact that we are *personally* not ready to take vanished or vanishing cultural forms seriously. What about the ideas that women should not wear trousers; that young people should never talk to their elders unless addressed; or that it is improper to eat peas with a knife? We tend to hail their (relative) disappearance as progress, not as laxity of manners.

Elias describes the late medieval or early modern banquet as a scene of emotional intensity, intimacy and spontaneity. His most important source is *De civilitate morum puerilium* by Erasmus, a guidebook on manners that was widely read at the time. After its publication in 1530 it was almost immediately translated into major European languages (to English for the first time in 1536), and it was, for instance, printed in Swedish in 1620 and in Finnish in 1670 (and again in 1693). The long time span testifies to the cultural lag between the centre and the peripheries of Europe, but also to the continuing popularity of the original work. For many years it remained prescribed reading in schools, no doubt in part because of its good Humanistic Latin.

Readers of *De civilitate* may be surprised to find, among its many instructions about table manners, rules that any adult today would find self-evident. Erasmus tells his reader, for instance, not to lick his fingers or wipe them on his jacket, not to drop leftovers on the floor and not to help himself to all the best bits from the shared dish.[24] These are things we would only feel the need to point out to children. But then, why ever might that be – if not because Erasmus *did* write his book for children?

On the other hand, Erasmus also lists rules of polite behaviour that strike modern readers as either old-fashioned or as plain unintelligible. For instance, you are not to pass anything at the table with your left hand; not to stand with your legs crossed; you are enjoined to kiss the bread if it accidentally falls on the floor:

> If thou geue or turne any thing, take hede thou doe it not with the left hande.

> In Italie certaine menne for honor sake doe laie one foote uppon another, nor they sustayne not themselues but as it were uppon one legge, after the maner of storkes, if this gesture be côvenient for little children, I know not.

> Our elders in al repastes did eate bread with great reuerence as a holy thing: and of that commeth the custome of this time, to kisse the bred, yf perchance it bee fallen upon the grounde.[25]

The custom of kissing the bread survived almost down to modern times in parts of Eastern Europe, no doubt reinforced by the role of bread in the Communion.[26] On the whole, the associations with religion in *De civilitate* are numerous, which gives its descriptions of social life a characteristically ceremonial aspect. Grace is said before and after meat as a matter of course. Seating at table is strictly regulated. On the street, respect must be shown towards anyone higher in age, holiness or rank:

> Yf thou meete with anye man in thy waye the which for his age is venerable, or reverend for his holinesse or graue for his dignitye, or otherwise worthy of honor, looke thou remember to geue him place, to turne thee and to make him waye, puttynge of thy bonet reuerently, and somewhat bowing thy knee.[27]

Medieval and early modern men and women ate with their fingers and took meat from a shared dish – something that, on

Elias's interpretation, is turned to an indication of intimacy and informality.[28] Today, the only formal occasion that allows finger food is the cocktail party, but experience tells us that even then intimacy does not necessarily ensue (and when it does, the bar will usually be closing). Elias also points to the fact that medieval travellers were often expected to share the same bed at inns. We should not, however, assume that a given practical arrangement must always imply intimacy. What counts as intimacy must be understood in relation to what, in the situation at hand, counts as the usual and thus in some sense neutral and anonymous way of doing things. Sharing the same bed perhaps did not feel much different from sitting down on the same couch today. But in present industrial society, with a plate, a bed and a room of their own for everyone, new forms of personal distance *as well as* intimacy have been made possible.

Elias ate with a knife and fork and Erasmus with his fingers; but is it not imaginable on comparison that Elias and not Erasmus might strike us as the uncivilized one? It is possible that, on witnessing life in the time of Erasmus, it would strike us as utterly ceremonious. Many of our present forms of refinement were missing, but instead there were others we have lost.

The experience of cultural alienation would be reinforced if we were to travel in time to a pre-industrial peasant household. On visiting, the modern city-dweller would probably have violated a dozen unwritten rules before even sitting down for coffee. In the Finnish countryside, the kitchen-cum-living room was divided into a 'male' and 'female' hemisphere by a limit that would be crossed only exceptionally. The placement of 'male' and 'female' utensils followed the same pattern. Ethnologist Irja Sahlberg tells us regarding peasant households in Kimito (southwestern Finland):

An invisible boundary would go from the chimney to the gable, dividing the room into a 'distaff side' and a 'spear side', or in the vernacular, the inglenook [*spisvrån*] and the men's side [*karlssidan*] ... Women and children would take their meals by the lowly 'eating table' [*matstol*, 'meat stool'] in the inglenook on their own, while men would eat by the 'high table' or 'men's table' diagonally from the fireplace.[29]

Sociologist Kirsti Suolinna informs me that, even in the early 1980s, she was told off by the master of the house in Ylimuonio, up in the north close to the Swedish border, when she happened to seat herself on the wrong side of the coffee table. The table marked the boundary of the male and female sides of the room, in a household that was incidentally quite modern-looking.[30]

It is then not obvious that agrarian society before the industrial age was less disciplined than modern society. The final verdict will of course in part depend on *who* will be making the comparisons and what their perspective will be. If present practices are adopted as the norm, we easily get the impression that our ancestors were generally careless people and yet for some reason constantly pre-occupied with trifles. The 'trifles' at issue might, however, on closer inspection be recognized as forms of everyday refinement now lost on us. In a sense, both parties would be fully justified to see the other as a bunch of barbarians. If two cultures are *different*, both will by definition employ distinctions that the other culture is lack-ing, and thus both could accuse the other of sloppy standards. We have it on record that non-Europeans, who were of course 'primi-tives' in the eyes of European travellers of past generations, have frequently perceived Westerners as childish and undisciplined. Instead of assuming an upward line of progress we should be aware of more complex patterns of variation.

Campaigning for civilization

The available sources in themselves hardly account for the rather ambitious generalizations typical of modernization theories.

Why, then, is it seemingly so natural nevertheless to present the development of Western civilization as a continuous increase of discipline and self-restraint? It is hard to resist the impression that there is a *demand* for certain ways of interpreting the past; for some reason we apparently wish to think of ourselves as more disciplined, more rational, more anonymous and also as cleaner than our ancestors. Our ideas of modernity reflect not only material changes, but changes of our self-understanding – a process that of course also belongs to the development known as modernity.

It is not irrelevant at this juncture to consider some profound transformations of demography and consequently of living patterns since the end of the eighteenth century. In Europe and North America, people were increasingly concentrated in urban areas where they would live in constant proximity to strangers. They would also be exposed to the temptations of cheap liquor and prostitution. The great majority of dwellings would afford little space for saving various odds and ends, and there would be no undisturbed little place for performing nature's offices outdoors. Against this backdrop of everyday logistical problems, the new triumphs of science and industry were announced – the marvels of indoor plumbing and improved detergents. The outcome was both to make cleanliness based on order increasingly troublesome and, gradually during the 1800s, to provide good opportunities for cleanliness based on water. These changes necessitated a major change of mind set, and it is hardly surprising that the inculcation of this *new* form of self-discipline required sustained campaigning. Pure air, light and cleanliness to everyone![31]

It is part of this picture that Western public discourse, at least from the late nineteenth century onwards, reflected the realities of the two growing urban classes. Self-discipline was perceived specifically as a virtue for the bourgeois and for the organized workers, whereas the assumed filthiness of manners among peasants and aristocrats was enough to send them to the dung-heaps of history. Nordström, the author of *Filth Sweden*, outlined in 1938 his vision of the Swedish worker as the noble knight of the future: 'A nobility based on neither birth nor purse but on a single thing, alone with the power to raze to the ground the old walls between classes and estates: *cleanliness, absolute cleanliness*.'[32] Americans, lacking the European caste system and taking pride in their progressive mind set, were early to diffuse the idea of cleanliness as a mark of civility.[33] By the late nineteenth century, social reformers in all industrialized countries had embraced the connection between cleanliness, self-discipline and progress. Cleanliness *equals* self-discipline *equals* progress.[34] Commenting on this general trend, Katherine Ashenburg quotes a statement from 1923 to the effect that, without a daily bath, 'no one can be really clean, nor either feel or express Culture' – adding her own rider, 'So much for Michelangelo, Beethoven and Jane Austen.'[35]

Already somewhat earlier, administrators in many countries had started to campaign for the bourgeois virtues among the populace. In Scandinavia it was common practice to use the pulpit for such general information purposes before the spread of the newspaper. By the end of the nineteenth century, however, the civilizing agenda was mostly understood in terms of medicine and hygiene. Illness rather than sin was the thing to be afraid of in industrial society, and this was brought home above all to female members of the household. A Swedish handbook for housewives, *Kvinnans bokskatt* (The Woman's Book Treasure), informed them in 1913 that 'already a quite small number of harmful germs are enough to cause a so-called "infection", i.e. to enter the body and there give rise to harmful effects, viz. diseased conditions.'[36] The trend was the same in all industrialized countries, with the United States taking the lead. Susan Strasser points out that after the 1890s, whenever popular magazines discussed health questions in that country, the focus was primarily on germs and on the various ways in which germs might make contact with people.[37]

Yet the health issue was just the tip of an ideological iceberg. As the following excerpt from a Finnish writer makes clear, 'dirt' was perceived as a general state of licentiousness. 'Cleanliness', in contrast, signified self-control in all areas of life:

> 'Man is an animal', you cannot help exclaiming, when you see human beings in dirty dwellings, wearing soiled, sweaty garments or using substances not fit for human consumption. Human dignity is then gone, man has no understanding of his own condition, for *a human being* must without fail be externally tidy and clean, pure as to the body. Man is an animal also when he abuses intoxicating substances, when he in his drunkenness has lost all self-restraint and self-determination, when the powers of his soul are paralysed and, slave to his animal passions, he only follows their lead . . . Thus we must keep in mind that whoever wants to bear the name of *human being* must keep his home and his attire clean and also follow the requirements of cleanliness in his entire life, for otherwise it is fair to say that he is an animal.[38]

In other words: human beings are humans, but if they don't take care they turn into animals. A beast is not to blame for being a beast, but human bestiality is always a case of degeneration. 'Purity' above all implied keeping off liquor, but also sexual self-control. 'Self-abuse' (masturbation) was feared to the degree that sex with prostitutes was sometimes presented as the lesser evil.[39] Judging by alarmed letters by young readers to a popular journal around 1900, health risks had become the main motivating force in the struggle for sexual self-control.[40] Conversely, physical health and cleanliness were the best protection against licentiousness. 'Daily external lustrations of the tender parts of the body are an excellent remedy against moral dissolution, but only the pure in heart will go fully secure.'[41]

The well-documented problems of malnutrition, overworking, inadequate housing and filth would above all be tackled with the help of education, which in the beginning was strongly dependent on charitable work by individuals. One example was Annie Furu-hjelm, daughter of a Finnish admiral in imperial Russian service, who spent the winter of 1892–3 in the northeastern backwoods of Finland in order to organize an asylum for children from destitute families. She was astonished to find that 'the common people in the region are reported never to flog their children – they are allowed to grow up in complete liberty.' That would of course change in the new institution, where 'human beings' would be made out of them.[42] Another thing to change would be the attitudes concerning dirt, for, according to then still prevailing local wisdom, 'Cleanliness, that's what kills you off.'[43]

Meanwhile in the industrialized heartlands of Europe and North America, after roughly 1850 'urban squalor' became a set topic for fiction and non-fiction alike. Typically, bourgeois debate on sanitary problems in the cities focused on unsound conditions in the home, not in the workplace. Accordingly, urban planning and education (of workers and their dependents, not of employers and slumlords) were perceived to be the chief remedies. The equation was *Cleanliness = Self-discipline = Progress*. Cleanliness was enlightenment, responsibility, health, modesty and light. Dirt was superstition, sloth, sickness, excess and darkness.

The interesting thing about this equation of the campaign for civilization was that it worked very well in both directions. It meant not only that the spiritual achievements of a person could be read off from the condition of his or her clothes and armpits, but that a person of supposedly low cultural level was designated as filthy and slovenly. What this might mean in practice is highlighted by Susan Strasser. She cites a 1906 survey of the sanitary situation in American cities, with the author deploring the 'careless and filthy class of waste' collected in high-immigration neighbourhoods. Those were areas populated by 'the least educated of the Russians, the Poles, Scandinavians, the Italians, and the Jewish element.'[44] The bad quality of waste from these areas was supposedly due to the generally careless way of life of the inhabitants, but Strasser points out that the opposite rather seems to have been the problem. The poverty-stricken inhabitants had *carefully* made sure not to throw out anything that might still be saved or used as fuel. The remainder was difficult to incinerate and hence 'filthy' in comparison with the unsorted refuse collected from affluent areas.

In this case, immigrant populations saw the very result of their industriousness turned against them as a marker of their backwardness. Historian David Ward describes a comparable phenomenon that Strasser also quotes.[45] In literature on urban misery, the scene of clothes lines hung between blocks of flats became the dominant visual symbol of dirt and disease. This sight of course existed precisely *because* of cleaning efforts by working women, but class prejudices made even 'images of cleanliness [appear] as portraits of squalor'.[46] Clothes lines were not visible in upper-class neighbourhoods whose inhabitants sent their laundry to washerwomen and commercial cleaners. In sum, the equation of the campaign for civilization worked excellently from the point of view of those in secure possession of the trappings of civilization, for they were given the power to define others not only as uncivilized but as filthy.

The thesis of modernization

It is above all our *expectations* that make men and women of the past (all of them, all the time) appear filthy, impulsive and 'natural' in our eyes – for good and ill. In practice, Norbert Elias has worked out lingering popular images of the 'wild' world of the medievals, thus exploiting the 'Dark Ages' as a romantic foil to set off 'modern' phenomena to be scrutinized.[47] The result is a theory of civilization that, in the manner of nineteenth-century evolutionism, classifies certain cultures as more primitive than others.[48] 'Primitive' is, to be sure, not only a term of abuse, as it also carries associations of living in close contact with nature and with true unspoiled human essence. Reflections on medievals and savages can be employed as vehicles for criticism when contemporary development is perceived as unnatural, thus tackling a pressing issue of our time: the contrast between the human being as part of nature and as agent of civilization.

A major function of our representations of the 'pre-moderns' is to serve as building-blocks of *contemporary* self-understanding. This is most easily noted when our schematic images lead to absurdities. Suppose again, with the description cited from Lyttkens, that pre-moderns were constitutionally unable to make any clear distinction between themselves, their families and the physical environment, which supposedly implied that at meals, there was no sharp boundary to be drawn between human hands and the food.[49] Did the pre-moderns chew off parts of their hands by mistake, never noticing the difference? Did they confuse their own names with those of their family members? The answer is that these descriptions are not meant to be taken literally, for the real message is about *our* self-understanding. It is about us, as members of a culture defined by ideas of individuality, rationality, discipline and human dominion over nature.

Thus the celebration of the abject in contemporary thinking about culture is, I believe, born out of a need to challenge the Enlightenment view of progress. But it also appears that the very project of vindicating our natural filth still carries some philosophical baggage from Enlightenment metaphysics. Dirt, which is conceived of as symbolic and thus in a sense an arbitrary category, is implicitly contrasted with a background of *material reality*, understood as a domain of pure science ultimately outside unaided human perception. We should now turn to look at this idea of 'matter'. In the theoretical discourse, dirt is typically perceived as a very strange thing, to be banished to the misty regions of symbolism. I believe this is because *matter* is not perceived as strange enough.

PART III

SETTLING ACCOUNTS WITH MATTER

This world is *difficult*. The notion of difficulty here is not a reflexive notion which would imply a relation to oneself. It is out there, in the world, it is a quality of the world given to perception (just as are the paths to the possible goals, the possibilities themselves and the exigencies of objects – books that ought to be read, shoes to be re-soled, etc.), it is the noetic correlate of the activity we have undertaken – or have only conceived.

Sartre, *Sketch for a Theory of Emotions*[1]

And can any of you by worrying add a single hour to your span of life? If then you are not able to do so small a thing as that, why do you worry about the rest?

Jesus (Luke 12:25–6)[2]

NINE

Between Facts and Practices

The very nature of the relationship between ourselves and
what is external to us, a relationship which consists in a
reaction, a reflex, is our perception of the external world.
Perception of nature, pure and simple, is a sort of dance;
it is this dance that makes perception possible for us.

Weil, *Lectures on Philosophy*[1]

Dirt as a problem, once more

What is 'dirty'? What happens when an object is classified as dirty?
Looking back to the previous discussion, at this point it is possible
to think of two opposite approaches to the question.

There are, firstly, various versions of reductionism, holding that
human consciousness takes in an originally neutral reality in a
selective and fragmentary manner. The human being comes to
classify parts of the world as impure in accordance with her intellectual and emotional needs, but her classifications are, logically
speaking, arbitrary: humans might in principle one day just start
applying some completely new set of categories to the world. The
second approach, opposed to reductionism, would imply naive
realism of a kind, presenting dirt and soiling as real qualities of
the world. They are qualities to be found out there, quite independently of any human tendency to classify them as such. We call
things dirty simply because they *are* so.

The latter conception, at least in the form just presented,
might strike the reader as exceedingly naive, and that is of course

why I have called it *naive* realism. At the same time it is hardly a coincidence that we recognize exactly this position as the 'naive' one. It represents an unreflective attitude, but one that in some ways strikes us as the natural default position before reflection sets in. But if philosophical analyses of our relation to dirt really aim to describe our concepts as they are – and not, for instance, to replace them with better ones – then the natural attitude should be the obvious starting point for any description, even though it does not have to be the end point. In *some* sense, then, we must accept the naive idea of a world where dirt really exists.

We must do so, but the question is whether we are philosophically entitled to do so. This conundrum depends on the presumed impossibility of attributing meaning and purpose to objects. Unlike a *subject*, an 'object' seems by its very definition to be something passive and lifeless. The world conceived apart from consciousness is, according to the philosophical majority view, colourless, devoid of purpose and, so to speak, motivationally inert. This amounts to a kind of 'duplicity in the comprehension of the material world', as described by Tim Ingold:

> On the one side is the raw physicality of the world's 'material character'; on the other side is the socially and historically situated agency of human beings who, in appropriating this physicality for their purposes, are alleged to project upon it both design and meaning in the conversion of naturally given raw materials into the finished forms of artefacts.[2]

To use a frequent phrase in this context (originally from Max Weber), the modern world is supposedly 'disenchanted' in comparison with the meaningful, teleological, divinely created reality inhabited by our ancestors. Applying this point to our present theme, the philosophical problem of how to understand the dirty and the clean is a consequence of our generally double-minded relation with the material environment. In our heads we no longer believe in the enchantment of the world, but our hearts and bodies still *live* it. The task at this juncture is to see how to make sense of the unreflexive view.

Fetishism

Anthropologist Arjun Appadurai navigates amid these difficulties in an essay on commodity exchange. He asks the question, 'what makes an object *valuable*?' 'Value' is not a physical concept and so the question is how physical objects may possess it in the first place. Appadurai argues, however, for 'the conceit that commodities, like persons, have social lives'.[3] He is critical of what he describes as '[c]ontemporary Western common sense':

> Though this was not always the case even in the West . . .
> the powerful contemporary tendency is to regard the world
> of things as inert and mute, set in motion and animated,
> indeed knowable, only by persons and their words.[4]

The author calls for a reassessment of the modern theoretical consensus and a return to something like the attitude Marx described as the fetishism of commodities.[5] Appadurai argues that there is something to be gained by treating things as valuable in themselves; as having value independently of any human act of conferring value to them:

> Even if our own approach to things is conditioned neces-
> sarily by the view that things have no meanings apart from
> those that human transactions, attributions, and moti-
> vations endow them with, the anthropological problem is
> that this formal truth does not illuminate the concrete,
> historical circulation of things. For that we have to follow
> the things themselves, for their meanings are inscribed in
> their forms, their uses, their trajectories. It is only through

the analysis of these trajectories that we can interpret the human transactions and calculations that enliven things. Thus, even though from a *theoretical* point of view human actors encode things with significance, from a *methodological* point of view it is the things-in-motion that illuminate their human and social context. No social analysis of things (whether the analyst is an economist, an art historian, or an anthropologist) can avoid a minimum of what might be called methodological fetishism. This methodological fetishism, returning attention to the things themselves, is in part a corrective to the tendency to excessively sociologize transactions in things, a tendency we owe to [Marcel] Mauss, as [Raymond] Firth has recently noted.[6]

Appadurai rejects real 'fetishism' as incompatible with the 'formal truth' that inherent value is impossible from a 'theoretical' point of view. But he argues that, even though objects in reality have no value in themselves, in practice anthropologists need to approach them *as if* they had value. Otherwise it would in many cases be impossible to understand why people *want* to own them. From the point of view of the agent, things are valuable not because they are traded or bought and sold at a price, but instead they *are* bought and sold because they are valuable. For this reason, Appadurai wants to hold on to a view he describes as *methodological* fetishism.

Why does he believe 'real' fetishism must still be rejected? Appadurai assumes this is self-evident. He apparently thinks it follows from logic: the *concept* of a physical thing or object is simply incompatible with the idea of inherent value. There is a philosophical term for the kind of logical contradiction he seems to have in mind (even if he is not using the term here). To ascribe a thing inherent value would involve absurdity of the kind known as a 'category mistake'. To say that physical things might have inherent value comes across as something like saying that squares might be round. One might say: the *concept* of a square rules out roundness and the concept of a physical thing rules out inherent value.

If that indeed is true, what now about 'methodological fetishism'? Appadurai argues that we nevertheless, in research, must act *as if* things had inherent value. My question is whether this kind of split between theory and method is intelligible. Can we really 'act as if' a logically contradictory idea was true? For instance, can we act as if a square might be round? Can we act as if physical things had inherent value if we think that that is logically impossible? Appadurai thinks we can and, in practice, must.

The problem with this, as I see it, is this. A logically impossible state of affairs is not merely ruled out. To say that it is logically impossible is furthermore to claim that we cannot even coherently think what it would be like for it to be true. If round squares are logically impossible we cannot imagine what a round square would be like; and hence we cannot act as if there might be round squares. Similarly, if it is logically impossible that physical things might have inherent value, then we cannot imagine or act as if they had any. In sum, if 'real fetishism' is ruled out as logically impossible, then Appadurai's 'methodological fetishism' must also be so. Conversely, if methodological fetishism is possible, then real fetishism will also be so. My suggestion is this: we should not simply assume that these issues have been settled above our heads by 'Logic', but we should confront different ideas and see under what circumstances we might make sense of them.

Let us discuss round squares. I might point out to you that there are several round squares in the world, with Tahrir Square in Cairo and Place de l'étoile in Paris among the most famous ones. 'Well, yes,' you respond, 'but this wasn't what I meant by "square". What I was saying was that squares in the *geometrical* sense cannot be round.' In telling me this, you would be highlighting the fact that you and I share a practice, Euclidean geometry, and within *that* practice there is no meaningful use for a certain expression ('round square'). Now consider the statement 'An *object* cannot have inherent value.' Also here it is possible to specify an intellectual practice within which the statement is true; namely that of Western physics from Galileo onwards. In other words, we say that (apart from measurement 'values') 'value' is not a physical concept, basically because teleology has no place in physics. But physics is not the only context where we encounter the idea of an object or a thing. Would we even say it is the most important one? No need to settle that question here, but in any case it is obvious from Appadurai's own description that it is *possible* for us, in certain contexts, to think of objects as inherently valuable. Right or wrong, it is not ruled out in advance by 'Logic'.

A collector might be desperate to add a certain antique to his collection and might be firmly convinced of its value. Does he want it because it is valuable or is it valuable because he wants it? In this case, there is no need for the *outside observer* to differentiate between the fact that he wants it and the presumed fact that it is valuable: it is enough to apply the formula that whatever is wanted is valuable, or –

> The value of a thing
> Is just as much as it will bring.[7]

On the other hand, from the *collector's* point of view the relationship is the reverse. The piece is not valuable because he wants it, but he wants it because it is valuable. It is also possible to imagine situations where genuinely valuable pieces are stowed away in attics or thrown on rubbish heaps with no one wanting them. Here one might then turn the tables and, with Göran Torrkulla, take up the position of a collector, adopting the passionate interest which is

> an expression of the ability, which we all share, in the most general sense to *appreciate* things in our environment, but also a *corrective* to artificial academic attitudes of

detachment or to our often merely half-hearted involvement, something that should not only give us food for thought but also make us ashamed of ourselves.[8]

The question of what the right attitude to take is must depend on the situation and on the kind of interest that one takes in it. It is, for instance, possible to criticize someone for taking an exaggerated interest in material possessions, just as it is possible to criticize them for neglecting their material environment or for failing to appreciate the beauty of it. Le Corbusier, in his plea for simple, functional interior design, chastised the prevailing tastes for 'pandering' to our avarice and creating a 'cult of the souvenir' to mask the cowardice and carelessness of not throwing away what is no longer of use.[9] His attitude is quite different from Torrkulla's, but he, too, thinks of our relation to objects as a moral one – in this case, as one that often includes false sentimentality and failure to distinguish between the beautiful and the ugly. In research, on the other hand, finding the best theoretical analysis is a methodological question to be solved from case to case by anthropologists, economists and other scholars. At this juncture, it is enough simply to state that the idea of teleology in material things is not immediately to be dismissed as *contradictory*.

Thing and object

But still, how can objects contain meanings? The idea that some kind of contradiction must be involved here is due to the underlying idea that an object – a shoe, a knife, an envelope – is essentially a collection of matter, and matter seems to be essentially devoid of meaning.[10] If the problem is described in this way, it looks as if only two answers were possible. *Either* our perception of meaning in the material world is an illusion after all, *or* meaning is in some half-mysterious way infused into the material world by something non-material. Neither solution strikes me as a happy one. What unites them is the unexamined assumption of there being a thing called 'what the material world *essentially* is'.

I would agree that material things are physical objects or, to put it differently, that they have physical qualities. But to say this is not yet to say much. For what is it for a thing to 'have physical qualities'? *Having* physical qualities is not one *more* attribute of a thing, but rather it means that the thing in question is a possible object of physical investigation; in other words, that certain kinds of question can be meaningfully asked about it. It is meaningful to ask about a knife, but not about a telephone number, what material it is made of: this indicates that a knife, unlike a telephone number, is a physical object. Similarly if we want to know how *long* the knife is we can use a measuring rod, but the length of a number (being an abstract object, not physical) is counted in digits and not in inches.

In *Philosophical Investigations*, Wittgenstein considers the statement 'Every rod has a length.' It is not an empirical discovery – it is not that every rod we have checked so far has had a length – but what Wittgenstein calls a 'grammatical proposition'.[11] A rod (as opposed to a sphere) is something of which we say it has a length. This is not only an observation about how we refer to rods in speech, but also involves the fact that we utilize rods for measuring distances. In this way, 'having a specifiable length' is not a *quality* of rods but more like a requirement that we make on rods, and the requirement itself is a feature of our practical engagement with them. That the material environment, as we might say, has geometrical qualities means that we can meaningfully engage with it in ways of this kind. It presupposes stability in the environment (so that things do not change their shape in unexpected ways) and it presupposes stability in us, together with our measuring rods. Similarly, saying that the world in which we live is 'physical' is simply to say that it is meaningful to ask physical questions about (many) objects, which includes undertaking certain kinds of measurements and investigations. On the other hand, that the material world is physical does not imply that physics exhausts the questions that might be asked about material things.

Here it is illuminating to consider the concept of a physical object. What kinds of practical engagement are implicit in this concept? In English, the expressions 'object' and 'thing' are used almost interchangeably, but it is possible to find a certain difference of emphasis. On the whole, 'object' is the preferred word when objects are discussed in the abstract or in a scientific context, while 'thing' often stands for tangible, ordinary objects – for instance, when anthropologist Tim Ingold, in his book *Making* (2013), makes use of a systematic distinction between 'things' and 'objects'. To treat a table, a cereal bowl and a milk jug as things instead of objects is to bring them into a relation with one another. They relate to each other via the activities of breakfasting, which establish 'a kind of choreography for the ensuing performance that allows it to proceed from the moment when you sit down to eat'.[12] Ingold further discusses Heidegger's essay on *The Thing* (*Das Ding*). The philosopher identifies the difference between object (*Gegenstand*) and thing (*Ding*), first of all, in terms of independence: a thing 'stands forth' as self-supporting whereas objects are only identified 'over against', or in relation to, the subject to whom they *are* objects.[13] Moreover, a thing involves nearness and it has a 'gathering' function by which it becomes a focal point in a world inhabited by human beings.[14]

In his essay, Heidegger uses the word *Gegenstand*, in the context plausibly translated as 'object'. However, German distinguishes not only between *Gegenstand* and *Ding* but also between *Objekt* and *Gegenstand*, with the former having an abstract sound and the latter more concrete and quotidian. Thus the right translation for *Gegenstand* might in other contexts be 'thing'. For my own part I have not tried to be systematic about when to write 'object' and when to write 'thing', because it seems to me it is just too late to do anything about existing usage – and even less, in the manner of Heidegger, to hark back to presumed original meanings. The distinctions at issue can be made in other ways. It might be said, of a particular thing, an ordinary object or *Gegenstand*, that it is 'an object-in-the-stream-of-life'. By *identifying* a jug as a milk jug and not just generally as a hollow object we implicitly fit it into an imaginable context of engagement. Conversely, disagreement and uncertainty about how to identify some object indicate difficulties of some kind about finding the right context for it. An object we cannot recognize at all has fallen on one side of the stream of life, so that it has now become a 'mere' physical object.

Theoretical science deliberately operates with 'mere' objects, because the everyday contexts of use for objects are simply not of any interest in scientific descriptions. What we need to see here, however, is that the scientific concept of a physical object is an abstraction made for theoretical purposes. It belongs to scientific theory, but this by no means indicates that material things are really, essentially or primarily, 'mere objects' in this sense and only afterwards given a 'subjective colouring' of meaning.[15] Rather it appears that it is possible for human beings to adopt (at least) two kinds of stance towards the environment, making the physical environment stand out either as a collection of neutral physical objects or as a network of meaningfully connected, concrete things. In the latter perspective, objects not only have teleologies but in a certain sense they are defined by their teleologies. To consider an example: a rotten egg may be described in terms of chemical analysis. But for our understanding of what kind of an object it is, it is also central that it exists in a continuum in time, defined through the opposition between an implied ideal state (a fresh egg) and a deviation from that state.

Which of these two ways of encountering the environment – as 'things' or as 'objects' – is the *right* one? At this juncture, it no longer seems to me to make sense to ask, as a *general* question, whether we have the 'right' to ascribe teleologies to things. To say that things 'have' teleological qualities is simply to say that our engagement with them occurs under the aspect of purpose and meaning. Rather than asking whether such qualities really exist, we should ask under what circumstances teleologies unfold and how they enter our relations with objects. My analysis is this: the teleology of 'lifeless' objects both depends on us and is independent of us. On the one hand, we breathe life into things through our engagement with them; on the other hand, we enter the scene only in Act Two. As human beings, we make our appearance in a world where objects always already have purposes, waiting for us independently of any ideas *we* might have. In the everyday experience of any single individual, ordinary objects are purposeful as a matter of course.

Place and space

In his early work, notably in his 'Theses on Feuerbach', Karl Marx made an attempt to diagnose philosophical problems connected with perception of the external world. He recognized them as inherent in the variety of philosophical materialism typical of the time (and advocated by Feuerbach, the target of his philosophical attack). The weakness of materialism, as Marx saw it, was that it did not 'comprehend sensuousness as practical activity' but only as a relation where an external and independent world of objects was mirrored in the mind of a 'contemplating' subject.[16] On the other hand, the important contribution of philosophical Idealism from Marx's point of view was its insight that the mind is not merely a clean slate taking in impressions from the outside. The mind has a hand in the creation of the world that it perceives. The external world is produced by it in the sense that the subject must perceive reality in accordance with its own cognitive structure. To gain knowledge of reality is to get acquainted with reality, which means getting engaged with it. But Marx voiced the complaint that the Idealists, even though they understood this, had only developed the issue 'in the abstract', neglecting 'the real activity of sensing as such'.

The general philosophical situation has changed in the intervening 170 years, in particular because Absolute Idealism, one of the two main objects of Marx's scrutiny, is no longer around as a dominant academic philosophy. On the other hand, materialism of the kind that he was critical of is still widely professed, typically under the headings of 'naturalism' and 'scientific realism'. In his *Theses*, Marx wrote:

> The main problem with all Materialism up to the present (that of Feuerbach included) is that the concrete thing [*der Gegenstand*], reality, sense experience, are conceived only in the form of *the object* [*Objekt*] or of *contemplation*, not as *human activity of sensing*, as *practice*; not subjectively. This is why the *active* aspect was developed in the abstract, not by Materialism but by Idealism – which of course does not recognize the real activity of sensing as such. Feuerbach wants sensuous objects, really distinct from thought-objects; but he does not conceive human activity itself as an activity *directed* at concrete *things* [als *gegenständliche* Tätigkeit].[17]

In this paragraph, Marx changes the philosophical scene by no longer presenting the opposition between Idealism and Materialism in terms of ontology or the question of what kind of stuff (mind or matter) reality is made of. He frames the main contrast instead in terms of an active versus passive relation to the environment, opposing his own 'dialectical' materialism to traditional 'contemplative' materialism.[18] In engaging practically with the environment the human being re-creates it in her own image in two ways: in the sense that she introduces changes into it according to human needs *and* in the sense that her conception of external reality is formed as a result of her engagement with it. In accordance with the principle 'My relation to my environment is my consciousness,'[19] the central concepts are that of *the human being* standing in relation to nature and that of practice or *praxis*, understood as active engagement. These concepts together present the human environment at the same time as both objective (that is, independent of human thinking) and subjective (that is, a result of human consciousness). In 'Theses on Feuerbach', this new take on material reality is indicated in the contrast between 'object' (*Objekt*) and 'concrete thing' (*Gegenstand*), a contrast that presents certain difficulties to the English translator.[20]

Not unlike Marx, but also drawing on related ideas from Heidegger and Wittgenstein, Norwegian philosopher Jakob Meløe presents a similar dialectic in his discussion of the concept of *place*. In his essay on 'Places' ('*Steder*') he asks what constitutes something as a place.[21] Meløe operates with various examples. Geometrical space may in principle be divided into any number of areas of arbitrary size, which is why the mathematical reply to the question 'How many places are there on this chessboard?' would be 'As many as you like.' A chess player, however, would answer: 'Sixty-four quadratic fields, neither more nor less.' The answers are arbitrary so long as nothing is implied about why the question is posed, but as soon as we enter the practice of chess there is only one correct answer.

Meløe dedicates a further analysis to the concept of *harbour* among Norwegian fishermen. In the essay 'The Two Landscapes of Northern Norway', a harbour is described as a structure, natural or man-made, where land meets water. Depth, ebb and flow, qualities of the sea bottom, the prevailing winds and other circumstances combine with the qualities of the vessel to determine whether a place counts as a harbour. You can discover a natural harbour, but you can also be mistaken about it, which indicates that the harbour is in some sense there independently of human opinion. Yet at the same time, the *concept* of a harbour is dependent on a particular form of life: a life that involves seafaring vessels too large for their crew to draw ashore. In a world without such life there would be no harbours, just as there will be no *shelters* in a world where no one seeks shelter.

It is only within (the world constituted by) this practice that this slice of matter (wherein a slice of liquid stuff has been adjoined to a slice of solid stuff) will present itself as one object, that is, as this harbour. Its manner of presentation derives from this practice. The method of investigating *the concept of* a harbour, therefore, is this: Situate yourself within the practice that this *object* belongs to, and then investigate *the object* and *its* contribution to that *practice*. If an object belongs essentially to a practice, as a harbour does, and a hammer, a coin, a cheque, a king's sceptre, etc., then the concept of that object is our understanding of that object's contribution to the practice within which it is that object.[22]

This passage does not use the word 'thing', but the author obviously has in mind what Marx, Ingold and Heidegger would call 'things'. Neither the practice, nor the object or thing that contributes to the practice, must be let out of one's sight. The object or thing is individuated by the concept, which is constituted by the practice. In offering these descriptions, Meløe wants to illuminate Heidegger's related concept of *Zeug*, translated as 'useful thing' or 'equipment'.[23] Meløe's important example is the fishing boat, which receives its meaning via its participation in a functional practice, while also contributing to shape that very practice:

This example is an example of how the world receives places and forms through our activity in the world. It is also an example of how we cannot describe our activities in the world without also describing the world in which we are active. And it is an example of how our activities in the world provide our language with concepts, such as a place to call at [with a boat].[24]

Meløe argues that, in describing the world, we make use of a number of concepts rooted in our activities while, at the same time, our descriptions of the activities themselves involve references to phenomena in the world. In this way, in describing an instance of equipment we must move on to describe the use of that equipment and further on to consider the form of the kind of world in which the equipment *is* equipment: 'For, by considering an instance of equipment . . . you will be led almost logically into considering the form of the world where it is equipment.'[25] A fishing boat *alone* – without fishing gear but equally also without the harbour and the fishing ground and the people who depend on it for a living – would lose its identity as a fishing boat.

At this point we should be on our guard against too superficial an understanding of the point that Meløe is making. Above all he is not making use of a distinction between appearance and reality, in which the way the world appears to us would be contrasted with the world as it essentially is. When a site is identified as a harbour within the framework of a seafaring life form, this does not simply mean that the seafarer has, for practical purposes, carved out certain parts of an underlying, independently existing space. *That* would be to assume the existence of an initially neutral world that the seafarer only later classifies with his concepts. And we would then face the question of how to identify that initially neutral reality. A coastline may obviously be described in a variety of ways, many of which, from the fisherman's point of view, might appear neutral or might indeed tell him nothing – for instance, when only concepts of geometry are used. Meløe's main point is, however, that even *neutral* descriptions are tied to situations and practices within which they *are* neutral; perhaps those of a surveyor or a clerk at the Land Registry. A given practice – for instance, land surveying or fishing – will *open up the world* in a certain kind of way for us. It will create a world that includes places and things that belong to the practice in question.

The lesson is not that we are all individuals, each enclosed in a world of his or her own making. The point is that various situations in life make a diversity of features of the world available to all of us. The world opens up its features and places to us according to the kind of life we live and the kind of interest we take in it. Geometry after Descartes presents places as points or areas in space. Ancient geometry, on the other hand, was still primarily conceptualized in terms of places and not in terms of abstract space – the Latin *spatium* signified distance between two places. Thinking of places and not of space may indeed be more apt in the current context of environmental issues, because it allows us to argue for the protection of entire milieus and habitats instead of specific living species or specific historical buildings. This highlights the importance of agreeing on how we are to understand the *telos* of a particular place.

A tourist on summer holidays, seeing a lake slowly fill up due to overfeeding, will look at it differently from the farmer whose field borders on it.[26] The tourist will want overfeeding to stop and the lake to be restored to its 'natural' condition. The farmer perhaps thinks of the growth of land as a 'natural', slow change that has been going on for decades. Manure is an alien, defiling substance for the tourist but not for the farmer, for whom it is a life-giving element. They will probably even think differently when they specify the geographical area in question. For the tourist, the lake itself is the centre of her activity, but for the farmer perhaps the field is the centre and the lake is a periphery. The tourist and the farmer in a certain sense live in different worlds. That does not, however, preclude mutual understanding. By learning more about the world of the tourist the farmer will learn to know the tourist. But note also another thing: by learning to know the farmer's world the tourist will learn more about what it is to stay as a *tourist* somewhere.

A world of experience

Perhaps it is possible to make this general statement: the world will always already, at least implicitly, be described as a 'lived' world of some kind or other. To identify properties of the environment implies understanding how they are embedded in the kind of life that lets precisely those properties present themselves. A *geometrical* world is defined in terms of spatial extension, and those concepts imply the idea of taking measurements. Measuring as a practice is part of a social context, but a context that presupposes the physical stability of objects, including our bodies as well as measuring tapes. Finally, 'physical stability' of the relevant kind is *defined* with reference to the measuring methods in use. Thus in order to understand what geometrical qualities are we must presuppose practices of taking measurements, *together with* a world that 'fits' our measuring practices. The important point is that the relationship between the property or object and the practice is one where they mutually define each other.

Turning to dirt and soiling: even if Douglas may be criticized on many counts, she is certainly right in pointing out that our experience of dirt is never an isolated phenomenon. To consider the world *sub specie sordis* is to enter a system, an experiential space which, in accordance with the dialectic sketched above, may be described from two kinds of perspective. A world where there are dirty and clean objects is, on the one hand, a world where certain characteristics belong to objects, thus *allowing* certain practices; and it is, on the other hand, one where our practices with objects are of such a kind that they make certain characteristics of objects *appear*.

To describe an object as dirty implies defining its role in a lived environment; thus the apparently simple philosophical question of whether soiling *really* exists in the world does not make sense as a general question. Inquiries of this kind should be restated in the form, '*under what circumstances* does it make sense to ascribe such-and-such qualities to some object?'

Dance of the body

'Situate yourself within the practice that this *object* belongs to, and then investigate *the object* and *its* contribution to that *practice*.'[27] In an investigation of dirt and soiling, literally to follow Meløe's advice would be to identify the practice that gives meaning to judgements about soiling. That is, however, not a negotiable route forward.

One important difference between the concept of soiling and the concept of a harbour is that harbours are associated with a rather easily identifiable range of activities, while that is not true of dirt, soiling and cleanliness. In this respect, the latter rather resemble the general concept of a *place*. It would be possible to imagine a world without seafaring and without harbours but not without places, except perhaps as a world where no one lives and no one ever does anything. And one could not, in a corresponding thought experiment, eliminate every practice that involves the concepts of dirty and clean and still expect to end up with a recognizably human way of life. The form of life that makes 'dirty' and 'clean' present themselves as qualities should rather be understood as one aspect of *many* practices (almost all practices, I am inclined to say), and this is precisely why it seems impossible to imagine a culture that has no conception of cleanliness at all. On the other hand, we may try to say more about how the concern for cleanliness enters as an aspect of our various practices.

Here it is illuminating to think of Simone Weil and her take on perception. In her *Lectures on Philosophy*, Weil develops the idea that human beings perceive objects via the responses that their human bodies give, which is why perception of the nature is 'a sort of dance'.[28] For instance, in carrying a large book with two hands we feel the book as a unitary object which requires our hands to move in tandem.[29] Now consider what is involved in cleaning the surfaces of a sink: the disgust at taking up a wet scouring cloth; drenching the surface with the cloth and scraping at ingrained stains with your nails; at the same time avoiding making mess with slops on your clothing. Wearing an apron allows you to move closer to the wet surface and to use your arms more energetically. Once done, you look with deep satisfaction at the result, breathing in the reassuring scent of detergent. Much of our relation to dirty surfaces is coloured by various reactions of attraction and repulsion. Apart from this kind of dance, our notion of dirt would simply be different from what it is. But the dance can also be seen from the opposite perspective, for it is also true that the dance has a kind of unity and order determined by its object, the removal of dirt. Actually existing dirt gives the attraction and repulsion their point, for otherwise your movements would be like a pantomime, a game of football without the ball, a christening without the baby.

A man walks restlessly in his flat, picking up books, opening them and putting them back, turning the waste-paper basket upside down, emptying drawers and shelves and quickly stowing everything back again. What is happening? It all makes sense if we know that he is looking for something. Moreover, his very pattern of movements is suggestive of the kind of object he is after: a receipt, a letter; not a balloon. The unity of the *object* gives the movements a meaning, the scarlet thread. The search follows a pattern because of the limited number of ways in which a receipt exists and *can* be lost, and for that reason checking the ceiling would not even constitute one possible part of the search.

Quite similarly, the proper methods of cleaning a sink are dependent of the kinds of way in which a sink *can* be soiled, and in that sense, soiling is a fact that explains the patterns of cleaning. On the other hand, there seems to be a difference. For it is also possible to say that what *counts* as 'soiled' is in part dependent on our reactions and on our existing methods of cleaning, which is why we cannot really define 'soiling' in abstraction from practices of cleaning. In contrast, it would *not* seem right to say we cannot define 'receipt' in abstraction from our methods of looking for receipts, even if it is certainly true that receipts are generally things that are kept in safe places and which may be lost and looked for. Whereas, if we were never to react to dirty objects and never wanted to clean them, we would not really have the idea of dirt at all as we now have it.

At this juncture we have met with a kind of dialectic which is not easy to solve; and in fact I believe we *should not* try to solve it. The one half of it implies that we cannot understand the meaning of 'dirty' and 'clean' without considering what we *do* with dirty and clean things, and thus these notions exist only in the lives of beings who react to their environment in certain kinds of way. The other half of the dialectic says that we cannot *describe* those reactions unless we presuppose an already existing contrast between dirty and clean.

The same chain of arguments can finally be employed to criticize the idea that judgements about soiling really just express human subjective (culturally or biologically engendered) feelings of disgust. The question to raise here is how we would identify and individuate the kinds of feeling that are at issue. How does the shivering feeling at picking up a dirty cleaning cloth differ from the feeling we get when we bite into aluminium? Both feelings can be described as ones of discomfort. An easy way to differentiate between them is of course to specify what the feelings are feelings *of*, but in that case we are no longer speaking of mere feelings but about the things that give rise to them. As previously, the circle of the argument closes itself; feelings of discomfort are a typical feature of our relation to soiling, but in order to specify what kind of discomfort this is we need to refer back to the fact of soiling.

Subjective or objective

Summing up, we get two conclusions. Firstly, dirt exists because certain attitudes and patterns of behaviour exist. Secondly, those attitudes and patterns of behaviour exist because dirt exists. My argument was that neither side of the coin should be explained away, for describing a world as dirty and clean and, on the other hand, describing *life* in a dirty and clean world, amount to the same thing. Dirt and soiling belong to a world that contains 'things' rather than 'objects', even though this is not to say that only things can be dirty; also people, animals and plants can be.

But perhaps the reader is still under the impression that there is a question unanswered: do objects objectively have teleologies and 'thingness', or is this simply something that human beings read into objects? At this point I must simply hope that the question no longer appears relevant to anyone who has followed my reasoning. For the central aim was precisely to dissolve the question in this general form. As perceiving subjects, our perception and judgement depend on the one hand on subjective aspects (such as human anatomy, our culture and our historically specific individuality) and, on the other hand, on objective aspects having to do with the character of the objects that we encounter in perception. However, what this general distinction amounts to in specific situations is not at all self-evident. How do we distinguish in a concrete case between what belongs to the object as such and what is an addition by us? At this juncture, it is no use to take up positions in an already existing war of attrition between realists and antirealists, a conflict that has produced much heat and confusion in the philosophy of science. Compare here with two further entries from the 'Theses on Feuerbach':

> The question whether objective truth can be attributed to human thinking is not a question of theory but is a *practical* question. Man must prove the truth, *i.e.*, the reality and power, the this-sidedness [*Diesseitigkeit*] of his thinking, in practice. The dispute over the reality or non-reality of thinking which is isolated from practice is a purely *scholastic* question ... All mysteries which lead theory to mysticism find their rational solution in human practice and in the comprehension of this practice.[30]

If I understand Marx correctly he is not telling us: forget about objectivity; let's do something practical instead – how about a revolution? But it is not very far off the mark to paraphrase him as saying: the concepts of reality and truth do not stand for metaphysical entities but they are *thinking tools* for problem-solving. It is hardly even possible to imagine serious thinking that is not truth-oriented in some way or other; that is, we cannot imagine thinking that has no use at all for distinctions between the real and the merely apparent or imaginary. To say *that* is one thing; it is quite another to claim that all our questions about reality mechanically apply the same, one and unchanging distinction.[31] The general point that thinking aims at truth does not get us very far unless we work out its applications in specific areas of human thought and action. Similarly, the point that true beliefs accord with reality must be supplemented with an understanding of *what it is*, for a particular belief in a particular context, to accord with reality or fail to do so.[32] That is, we must be able to situate it in a system of practices.

The distinction between clean and dirty is then, if you like, a *real* distinction once a certain relation is in place between human beings and the environment. However, in the context of philosophical debate, the phrase, 'a *certain* relation' in practice far too often stands for 'an *uncertain* relation' – that is, a relation that has still not been specified.[33] In what ways do human forms of life and engagement allow the world to unfold as clean and dirty? Adapting the language of metaphysics: what are the transcendental conditions of soiling?

TEN

To Dress and to Keep

The human being as anti-Midas

A dirty and clean world is above all a world where we *care* for things, and Heidegger had good reason to describe our basic relation to the environment as one of care, or of caring engagement (*Sorge*).[1] The easiest way to see the bearing of this point is to consider the opposite: the kind of world that resists our categorization in terms of clean and dirty. Think of unspoiled nature. I go for a walk in the forest; on the ground I see a bird's nest, a hare's droppings, decaying leaves. Suddenly there is a discarded rubber boot. It is refuse. It is dirty, covered with mud. But the muddy ground itself, the soil that ruins my shoes – is it dirty? And if it is, was it so already *before* I came here? At this juncture one would be tempted to say that pure mud, soil as it is and in itself, is made dirty only under the soles of human feet – an idea that turns human presence into a kind of negative Midas touch. In the words of Edwyn Bevan, 'in an uninhabited world moist clay would be no more dirty than hard rock; it is the possibility of clay adhering to a foot which makes it mire.'[2]

Still, we should not let our ideas run away with us, for – apart from the fact that not only humans, but many animals clean themselves and are disturbed by various forms of soiling – we must ask exactly why the possibility of human contact 'makes' a material dirty. Physical changes are involved in the process of soiling, such as when clay adheres to a surface, but clearly the crucial change must be understood in the light of teleology. Human (or conscious animate) presence is essential in the situation, for it invites a perspective on the environment as a meeting place between nature and non-nature. The crucial change, I suggest, consists in the introduction of possible *questions* that would have no application in conditions of untouched nature – for example, 'Can I walk here without ruining my shoes?'

Soiling and pollution may take place in meetings between nature and non-nature, for instance when a coastal area is polluted in an oil disaster. Nature itself also causes pollution by making contact with non-natural objects like clothing, shoes or buildings. The connection between the ideas of purity and of undisturbed nature is grounded in the combination of two circumstances:

1. 'Nature' constitutes the opposite of 'culture', thus encompassing those elements and influences in our environment that are neither caused nor controlled by human action – which certainly invites the question of whether there is any nature left on our densely populated planet; whether there are milieus that still carry no trace of human presence. However, naturalness must not be understood as absolute isolation from everything human. Rather, the usefulness of the concept of 'nature' lies in its contrastive effect. Nature – or rather, the natural – is an aspect of *human* environment, which implies that elements of our environment are natural *to the extent that* they are not created or controlled by us.

2. On the other hand, the primary master objects of soiling are exactly the kinds of thing which, in the framework of our material culture, may require human intervention. Objects present themselves as clean or dirty, and they are cleaned and protected from dirt, because they constitute worthwhile objects of caring engagement.

The two points combined present nature in juxtaposition with culture. Nature is described by definition as pristine and untouched and culture as necessarily preoccupied with protecting and restoring the cleanness of objects. Insofar as nature *is* nature it counts as untouched and, in *that* sense, as pure. Polluted nature is ruined *as nature* to the extent that it is polluted, just as nature tidied up and 'landscaped' is no longer nature. Apparently, our conceptions of nature and of pollution or soiling are two sides of a coin: *what* we would count as absence of pollution and soiling indicates, by the same token, what we would count as a 'natural' process in the environment under consideration.

The idea that dirt is absent in nature implies, in other words, not that nature is *clean* but rather that nature is *pure* and, in this pristine state, lies completely outside the contrast between clean and dirty. Purity reigned in Paradise, but not because of Eve's spring cleaning. Precisely for this reason, it is also possible to speak of soiling with euphemisms that assimilate it with a natural state of things instead of with human carelessness. Novelist Yury Tynyanov uses this imagery in his description of dirt roads in the vicinity of St Petersburg in Pushkin's time: he writes of the unpaved roads giving off 'blessed dust from the first moments of Creation'[3] – a turn of phrase that, in modern times, is echoed in the Ukrainian expression 'holy earth' (*sviata zemlia*), used for describing, for instance, a particularly filthy piece of clothing.[4] The core of this metaphor apparently comes from Genesis where, in the first days of Creation, certainly no cleaning was done but God could still see everything he had made and conclude, 'indeed, it was very good.'[5]

Responsibility

The purity of untouched nature implies that an object assigned exclusively to 'nature' cannot appear as a primary master object of dirt. It also seems counterintuitive to describe extremely large or diminutive objects – such as solar systems or atoms – as dirty. This appears to be connected with the impossibility of intervention. How would you polish an atom or a galaxy?

The role of physical distance between human being and object seems also to be important. Dirt and soiling can be relevant only within a certain physical range. When we are far away we cannot see, feel or smell the dirt, and when we close in on the object the dirt dissolves into its microscopic constituents. Here, of course, nearness and distance are not to be understood simply in terms of geometry but in terms of the appropriate distance for the kind of engagement that cleaning involves.[6] The effects of nearness and distance were demonstrated in a photo exhibition, 'Kitchen Dreams', that I happened to visit in my home town of Åbo.[7] The motifs on display included 'dried orange juice in glass', 'meat-dish of steel', 'ladle and fork' and 'dirty plastic dish'. By approaching the objects very closely but focusing the camera outwards, artist Vilppu Vuorela achieved a decorative effect of coloured surfaces. He told an interviewer:

> Vilppu was sitting in the kitchen, looking at dried orange juice, the greasy kitchen sink, the dirty plastic dish and the dusty lamp in the ceiling. – Suddenly they started to look beautiful. I let my gaze wander through the mess in the kitchen. I blurred the focus until the things behind the lens started somehow to look sweet, he tells us. In the pictures, dirt stains have transmuted into an almost unrecognizable, soft, beautiful shine. The sink and the plug glow in purple, the juice stain is like a floating planet or a ball of egg yolk making an escape.[8]

With the camera changing focus from close up to far out, the viewer's relation to the items is changed so that they all of a sudden cannot look dirty. The artist tells us that one morning he simply could no more face the unwashed dishes towering in the kitchen and, as a reviewer puts it, he took the kitchen door out of his Angst.[9] Creating a photo exhibition was his way of coping with his own (as he saw it) exaggerated perfectionism, the will to control.

Dirty objects may be living beings, their bodies or body parts (for example human beings, dogs, hair), household items (cutlery, tools, garments, furniture, photos), places and spaces for habitation and transport (houses and streets). Also work, occupations, habits and thoughts may be dirty. For most of the things just mentioned, it seems part of their definition that they are *someone's*: someone's hair, someone's home or someone's pet. The material things we own are built of atoms, but this is not to say that we own atoms. Things that do not belong to anyone – say, stagnant water in a pond; flies – are typically described as dirty only when they risk sullying something that does have an owner.

The important feature here is not legal ownership as such but the fact that things that may have an owner are also things of which someone – not necessarily a specific person, but still someone – is in charge. This 'someone' is required to protect the object or to restore it to an acceptable state. In the language of metaphysics: *the transcendental condition of dirt is responsibility*.

Consider the perhaps not unusual family scene:

She: 'A pretty sight in here!' (*Meaning: There is a mess, and you should tidy it up!*)

He: 'What do you mean?' (*Meaning: You do it if it troubles you!*)

Thus differences in judgements about cleanliness can be a matter of taking different views on whether someone is in charge – and who it is.

The stewardship of objects

Susan Strasser aptly speaks of our *stewardship of objects*, the mutual relation between objects and ourselves that might also be called the contract we keep with things.[10] Material culture without this sort of engagement is hardly imaginable, but according to Strasser it was particularly noticeable in pre-industrial, pre-consumer society:

> Throughout most of our history, people of all classes and in all places have practiced an everyday regard for objects, the labor involved in creating them, and the materials from which they were made . . . Everyone was a *bricoleur* in the preindustrial household of the American colonies and, later, on the frontier; saving and reusing scraps was a matter of course. Cloth, wood, and food could only be obtained by arduous spinning, weaving, chopping, sawing, digging, and hoeing, by bartering with other products of strenuous work, or by spending scarce cash.[11]

As Strasser notes, her description is in its essentials applicable everywhere that humans live in conditions of scarcity – which on the whole may be described as the normal condition of humankind. Consider, for instance, the description that Ningtsu Malmqvist gave, in 1979, of the flat where her sister was living in the Chinese city of Chengdu. She observed the absence of any kind of dustbin, due to the simple reason that 'apart from ashes from the oven there was nothing to throw away.'[12] No food was discarded and old shoes, bones, feathers, rags and so on were all bought up by itinerant merchants.

Thrift was economically sensible in pre-industrial society, but it also had – and has – a moral dimension. 'Waste' in Old and Middle English stood for 'desolate region', but when the alternatives 'wilderness' and 'desert' were introduced in Middle English, 'waste' started to indicate moral censure. As verb, 'to waste' means, among other things, laying waste, 'bringing an estate into bad condition by damage or bad husbandry' and, by extension, it now means 'not making the *best* use of something' – thus, as John Scanlan points out, connecting with the 'notion of stewardship that placed humanity at the service of the Almighty'.[13] In this, pre-industrial households could appeal to Genesis, where the Garden of Eden was given to humanity 'to dress it and to keep it'.[14] The obligation not to waste certainly tended to conflict with other human needs: for instance, with the need of rest.

A culture where the parents' old garments are remade for the children, where fish bones are boiled for glue, where throwing away is always a sign of bad housekeeping – people in such a culture have a different relation to things as well as to each other than do most readers of this book. A dress that you have made by your own hands, or one made for you by Aunt Edna, is not so easily thrown away as one that comes from an unknown sweatshop of an unknown country. Paper tissues like Kleenex represent the other extreme: artefacts expressly produced for throwing away.[15] Such 'non-objects' have not only introduced a new kind of cleanliness and freedom but, for a hundred years now, they have been gaining more and more territory, with Aunt Edna constantly yielding to Kleenex.

At the other end of the trajectory we can already imagine a world where *everything* is disposable: clothing, cutlery and homes, all made of plastic, cardboard and paper and thrown away after use. In a world entirely built of disposable products, the very word 'dirty' would change its meaning and simply be synonymous with 'used'; instead of cleaning, things would simply be disposed of. This thought experiment may, however, only be carried to an extent. There are practical limitations, for at least the factories for making disposable products would have to be durable, and the factories would need to be serviced and kept clean. But there would also be a logical limit to this disposable world, even supposing Kleenex were raining from the skies. The inhabitants of this world would still be durable and so they would at least have a use for the concept of dirt as applied to personal hygiene. But *that* kind of life would still be strikingly different from ours – alienating, if we can imagine it at all. It is sometimes claimed that what makes human beings *human* is the use of tools, a claim that is not completely true, for tool-like use of sticks, stones and similar items has also been observed in apes and birds. It is closer to truth to locate the birth of humanity at the point when humans started to *save* their implements for the next time, which implies the need to care for them.[16] In conclusion, there will be a place for Aunt Edna even in the world of the future.

Refuse and rubbish

Susan Strasser's historical descriptions make clear that *refuse*, as the undifferentiated category of whatever is discarded, is a relatively recent phenomenon. Before the onset of cash economy in the last couple of centuries there was (at least in Western societies) no general practice of throwing things to the rubbish. Labour and, especially in the countryside, room for storage were abundant but money was not. Consequently, all even remotely usable materials were saved for future needs. If nothing else, organic matter could always be collected on a dung-heap and later ploughed into the garden as fertilizer. Leftover materials were accordingly not 'refuse' but *specific* materials stored for secondary use.

In his study of the municipal handling of waste in Finnish cities and towns *c.* 1830–1930, historian Henry Nygård notes that refuse was still an exclusively urban phenomenon. Still in a manual from 1969 'it was implicit that no "refuse" existed in the countryside.'[17] Even in cities, the waste from privies was seen as a valuable resource: the interest shown in it 'did not chiefly depend upon problems of disposal but rather the opposite: it was felt that the city did not manage to deliver sufficient amounts of suitable fertilizer.'[18]

Historically, our attitudes towards objects have gone through modifications that may be traced via linguistic changes. Strasser observes that words like 'garbage', 'rubbish', 'refuse', 'waste' and 'trash' tend today to be used as synonymous expressions for any material discarded as worthless.[19] But this is a new development. Consider 'litter', 'trash', 'debris', 'garbage', 'scraps' and 'junk'. Originally each indicated a *specific* rest product saved for secondary uses. 'Litter' (from medieval Latin *lectus*) meant 'bed', such as hay used for bedding. 'Trash' stood for branches and twigs lopped off from trees, stripped leaves of sugarcane and so on, all to be used as fuel. The word may have a connection with 'thrash' and 'thresh', and so may originally have meant material obtained by threshing. 'Debris' (from Old French *débriser* – 'break down') was material broken down or broken off from something. 'Rubbish' is derived from 'rubble', or 'pieces of undressed stone', used especially as filling-in for walls. 'Garbage' originally meant 'offal', such as entrails of chicken, used as food for human or animal consumption. 'Scrap' was 'material produced by scraping', as when paint is scraped from a wall or, alternatively, things scraped together – bits and pieces from the yard or scarce resources from wherever available. 'Junk' stood for pieces (chunks) of cable, to be reused for fibre.[20]

Pre-industrial English thus had little use for an umbrella term for refuse but it had a wide range of terms for specific materials, variously related to what we today vaguely cover by the word 'refuse'. Etymologically, these terms seem mostly to refer either to the method of their production or to the actual activity of collecting them; thus the dominant relation with rest products was not that of discarding but of saving.

Analogous developments can be traced in other European languages – the meanings of words for rest products moving from the specific to the general and their focus from saving to discarding. Philosopher Cyrille Harpet describes the development of the French *déchet*, 'refuse'. Etymologically, *déchet* (from Latin *decido*) is associated with something falling off or falling down; for instance, shavings and fragments falling on the floor during work on wood, metal or fabric. Instead of the concrete sense of something falling off, further development in language laid stress on the character of the fallen material as something lost and unsuitable for further use, a transformation that seems to indicate change of focus from individual handicraft to industrial production. Michel de Montaigne used *déchet* in 1580 for 'loss in measure, value or weight', which may occur in the course of manufacture, storage or use. In 1611 the word was used to mean loss of social status or privileges, until it finally got its present meaning of 'matter discarded or put aside as worthless'.[21]

The German *Abfall* is a direct translation of *déchet*, and it has gone through a completely analogous development. Its literal meaning would be 'falling off or away'. The huge economic encyclopaedia by Johann Georg Krünitz, published in 242 volumes between 1773 and 1858, describes *Abfall* in the first instance as the inclination of terrain, pipes and channels necessary for the smooth flow of water. *Abfall* is further associated with decline, decay and deterioration: 'deterioration (*Verfall*) of business, trade and techniques, through which the fortunes of a tradesman decline and perish'. *Abfall* in the present sense of 'refuse' is finally mentioned among specialized terms, in use for instance in beekeeping, where it is defined as 'the rubbish (*Unrath*), or fragments of wax, collecting on the ground underneath the hive' – and 'among craftspeople', in whose technical vocabulary '*Abfall* means whatever falls off during work and goes to the rubbish (*Krätze*)'.[22]

The related Swedish *avfall* (*affall* in the old spelling) shows a parallel history traceable from the sixteenth century onwards. In the first complete Swedish Bible edition it had the religious meaning of 'fall from grace', while in contemporary historical work it meant 'deserting an ally'. It had the further meanings of 'decease' and of 'loss of status or worth'. *Affall* in the sense of 'material that falls off' seems to enter the language in the seventeenth century, for instance, in connection with leaves (1689), dung (1762), hair and unripe fruit (1815) and, as in German, sinking water level (1648). The concern with manufacturing enters in the eighteenth century, when *affall*, in analogy with *déchet* and *Abfall*, is associated with work processes resulting in fragments of material falling off, as with tree felling (1762), the sugar industry (1774) and the metal industry (1788).[23]

The focus in the twentieth century seems to have moved again, away from problems of industrial production to those of disposal.

In European law, waste is defined as any item transferred, as it were, from use mode to getting-rid-of mode. Thus in France, waste (*déchet*) is specified as 'any substance or object or more generally, any movable goods discarded by its possessor, or such that the possessor intends or is obliged to discard it'.[24] This is closely modelled on the relevant EU directive.[25] The law replaced one from 1975 where waste was described as '*abandoned* goods'.[26] The current EU law is that the original producer retains ultimate responsibility for waste disposal, although it is usually delegated to a private or public waste collector.[27] The law now also specifies that a substance has *ceased* to constitute waste when properly treated and recycled.[28] The term 'final waste' stands for the remaining part that cannot be recycled with current technology; this also implies that the status of waste may change with the development of new methods of treatment.

As things stand now, our use of the concept of refuse simply reflects our desire to *throw away*. But where is 'away'; when things go there, where are they thrown? 'Away' is neither a concrete place nor a specific distance. Not everything in a landfill is away – not the fence around it, not the adjoining buildings and not even the refuse itself, if it still waits for transport for incineration or recycling. But from the point of view of the person who has discarded it, refuse is now safely tucked away somewhere 'else'. What constitutes 'away', in other words, cannot be specified without reference to the agent for whom it *is* away. The notions of *refuse* and *away* belong together: to throw an item away is to cut off one's contact with it, to wash one's hands of it, whereby the landfill becomes a visible symbol of our thrown-off responsibilities.[29]

Our relationship with objects usually takes the form of mutual dependence. Things must work and they must be unscathed and whole. Conversely, they make demands on us. The window must be cleaned and the car must be repaired up until the point when they terminate their contracts with us, our stewardship ends and they go to the refuse. But as we have seen, in industrial societies it is all the more often the human agent who is the first to terminate the contract, after which, it is to be hoped, objects return to nature as earth or, recycled, acquire new identities.

Problem waste constitutes the well-known exception to this cyclical process. Every cultural effort to create a well-kept and pleasing environment also implies the exclusion of (ex)-objects and spaces. The cultural utopia of freedom from natural decay contrasts culture not only with nature but with heterotopia, with an elsewhere, the negative mirror image of cultured landscapes.[30] It takes the shape of industrial no-man's-lands of oil fields, arising from our need of energy, and of landfills, arising from our need of living space without waste. As a consequence, entire neighbourhoods located in that 'elsewhere' now literally drown in waste. In the words of Pia Maria Ahlbäck,

> The environmental importance of heterotopias thus lies in the fact that they can return what has been abandoned, often in an inevitably doubly dystopian form, because it was not wished for in the first place ... The very nature which had already been forgotten and was imagined to have been finally overcome makes itself known again, now in a more degraded and threatening form: emphasizing that it is not possible to escape it.[31]

Meanwhile we keep dreaming of a safe elsewhere, the ultimate repository of our most hazardous waste products.

Keeping things alive

In decisions to throw away, *usefulness* is only one of the factors to consider. People save the most curious of things while they throw away perfectly good stuff. The decision hangs on the question of how the object connects with one's own life. Perhaps it carries memories of significant others. Conversely, it goes to the rubbish when its significant connections are severed; the object carries no more life within itself. Sometimes the death of the owner is enough. Who wants an unknown person's false teeth or passport photo? What about an odd shoe or a postcard lost on the way to the pillar-box? In all these cases a thing turns to trash without any perceptible change occurring in the item itself. Something that was once in the middle of life, as part of some activity, is now left on one side while life is busying itself with something else. Conversely, the fight against precisely this kind of decay involves the striving to keep things alive.

Consider a typical feature of our use of functional objects: the rhythm of work and rest. Tools, and also things like jugs, cutlery, human hands and human mouths, are set to work by engaging them with some material or other. The employment of utensils and human external organs characteristically involves active use, cleaning and rest (storage) succeeding each other by turns. A painter's brush must be dipped in paint, a smeary substance otherwise to be avoided. If the condition of the brush is already at that stage construed as 'soiled', the implication is that the would-be artist is not doing art but simply ruining a canvas by smearing it with some wanton substance (not that the line may not sometimes be difficult to draw). In the normal case, however, the question of whether the brush needs cleaning will only be asked when the brush is temporarily freed of its primary use, for the sake of storage or because the artist wants to switch to a different pigment. Thus the question 'Dirty or not?' is, for certain kinds of functional object, dependent on the rhythmical alteration of work and rest. This is on the other hand not the case with objects not typically used for engaging with other materials; objects for which soiling is not part of their functionality. The fact that someone has just read a book, seen a painting or looked through a window does not imply that the object must now be cleaned 'after use'.

The relation between functionality and dirt also shows in our attitudes to personal hygiene. Annie Furuhjelm gives one such case from her travels in the Finnish northeastern regions. 'It is not dirt at all, it is clean soot,' she cites as the local peasants' response to anyone who might criticize the darkened faces of the children.[32] Furuhjelm agrees that it would be a natural point of view in a family living in a *rökpörte*, a house with an old-fashioned chimney-less stove, where the smoke was simply let out through an opening in the ceiling. Soot in one's face constituted dirt there no more than it did in the stove itself, but it *would* be dirt when there was a new situation – for instance, when the family dressed up for church on Sunday. Signs of daily living, natural and neutral as they were in the midst of ongoing activity, were removed in view of the approaching Sunday.[33]

The distinction between activity and rest also gives rise to typical, desperate tidying-up efforts when a visitor is expected. The point of such exercises is not necessarily to deceive guests with a false facade, for they also mark a break with the routines of the everyday. Toys and books lying around, conveniently in hand on floors and tables and contributing to the daily living space, are cleared out as a welcoming gesture. The nature of cleaning as an interruption of routine is one reason why cleaning carries all the seeds of a destructive power struggle: conflicts may arise in the family about who is to define the shared space. Various ongoing projects lie about in the house waiting for completion, and where one person sees a mess, the other sees a space where *life* is lived – which explains why the preoccupation with neatness and cleanliness sometimes comes out as hate of life itself, as a wish to eliminate signs of ongoing activity in the name of cleanliness and order.

A cosmic order

A clean and dirty world is one characterized by the human steward-ship of objects. In this sense our relation to dirt is connected with a view of the universe as *cosmos* in its original sense: an organized lawful whole with objects following preordained teleologies and the human being bearing responsibility for them. But it sometimes happens that the world refuses to comply. Things fall over and break, they wear down, they are lost – something that Wittgenstein in a manuscript describes as 'the cussedness of things':

> 'The cussedness of things'. – An unnecessary anthropo-morphism. We might speak of the *world* as malicious; we could easily imagine the Devil had created the world, or part of it. And it is *not* necessary to imagine the evil spirit intervening in particular situations; everything can happen 'according to the laws of nature'; it is just that the whole scheme of things will be aimed at evil from the very start. But man exists in this world, where things break, slide about, cause every imaginable mischief. And of course he is one such thing himself. – The 'cussedness' of things us a stupid anthropomorphism. Because the truth is much graver than this fiction.[34]

The truth, according to Wittgenstein, is 'much graver', because we are stuck with a world that does not work as it should. We might throw up our hands in despair but we do not give in, for this world is our home. We feel responsible for it, we care for it, and we know that at least some small part of it may be kept clean and in order. In the final reckoning, nature – meaning death and decay – always wins. But even if the natural decay of things cannot be arrested for ever, we can at least seek to steer the decay in particular directions. We clean things, salvage them and repair them and, at times, we throw them away.

ELEVEN

What Is Mine and What Is Someone Else's

'and the two shall become one flesh.' So they are no longer two, but one flesh.

Jesus (Mark 10:8)[1]

The human body as a borderline object

In philosophical treatments of dirt and pollution, the usual tendency is to prioritize personal cleanliness over the cleanliness of objects. Our concern with the latter is often described as something derived from the more primordial impulse of shielding one's own body against foreign substances. But in many cases it seems there are good reasons for the analysis to take the opposite course. Sometimes the need of *personal* hygiene is, on the contrary, a consequence of the need to protect external objects against soiling – as, for instance, typically in the case of washing one's hands. As a person and a body, I can take on the roles of both primary and secondary master object for dirt. When I think of myself as dirty I mostly think of the feeling of being unwashed, for instance with greasy hair; in this case my hair is the primary master object. But sometimes my hair makes the collar of my shirt greasy, in which case my shirt counts as the primary and my hair as the secondary object. Judgements about soiling in everyday situations are informed in various ways by the question of what it means to handle objects in a responsible and appropriate way.

My own body occupies a special position in such judgements. Insofar as it is correct to speak of my body as an 'object' at all it is because my body partakes of the same conditions as other material things. My body may be damaged; someone may be looking for me (my body) in a crowded room. Yet at the same time I am also the one *for whom* all other things are, or may be, objects. From my own point of view the relation between my body and other objects is not symmetrical, but rather my body and the place it occupies constitute the reference point or midpoint of indexical expressions (such as 'here', 'over there').[2] Whatever is 'here' is here because I am 'here'.

I wake up in the morning in someone else's bed in a completely unfamiliar environment. I don't know where I am, and I have also lost my spectacles. I start *looking* for them, but I will *not* start looking for myself – for even if I don't know where I am I at least know I am 'here'. My further orienting task will consist in finding out *where* my 'here' is. There is definitely something odd with this description: it borders on nonsense, language on holiday, and this fact above all demonstrates that I was using expressions whose real home is somewhere else. We are approaching the limits of meaningful talk about *objects*. From my own point of view I am not merely an object.

Ideas of agency and responsibility enter here almost by necessity. When I enter a state of soiling or defilement *I am* the object that requires cleaning; but I will also be the person responsible for cleaning the object which is my body. My body enters the picture in two ways. It is partly something that makes physical contact with (other) objects and may soil them. On the other hand, my need to wash may also express a self-conscious attitude where I focus on my body and the state it is in. Even though it is not true that I am always to blame if I am dirty – for in many situations it is simply impossible to keep clean – it is not something I can treat with complete indifference. Largely the same points are applicable if we consider my relations with someone *else's* body. I can hardly ever treat *someone else*, another person, as a mere object.[3]

Imagine observing a conspicuously unwashed person, probably homeless, in an otherwise well-organized shopping mall.

Your reactions might range from disgust to irritation to pity, or probably a mixture (pity being in this case a reaction to his disgusting state), but this mixture of reactions is testimony to the strong symbolic connection between dirt and moral failure. The Latin root *sord-* carries both hygienic and moral associations. The adjective *sordidus* is derived from the verb *sordeo, sordere* – 'to be unwashed or unkempt', but also 'to be despised' – and the adjective correspondingly has both the aesthetic sense of 'dirty, unclean, seedy', the moral sense of 'mean, corrupt' and the social sense 'obscure, despised'. These associations are not just coincidental facts about language, for they follow from what has already been said about dirt and responsibility. We naturally think of the unwashed person's sorry state as something that must be a *concern* for him or at least *should* be so. Even in our disgust we differentiate between people and objects.

But exactly the ethical dimension of hygiene opens up for an incredible variety of human reactions to soiling, ranging from tenderness to extreme cruelty. One particularly disquieting aspect of judgements about soiling has (justly) received attention in the research literature: the use of dirt as a tool of domination. The power to stigmatize others as unclean and untouchable, thus reducing them to total subjection, contrasts with the rare occasions where someone who is given such power refuses out of pure selflessness to make use of it.[4]

Being unclean

When are we unclean? The general answer is the same as in the case of other objects: either we (our bodies) have made contact with unwanted substances; or it is to be feared that our bodies transmit substances that would be unwanted on other objects. But this is not yet to say anything about what kinds of substance *are* unwanted. Most human activities are of the kind that cannot be sustained without the risk of uncleanness. To refuse everything that might make you dirty is to refuse life itself. It starts with metabolism. According to a newspaper report: 'A human being secretes roughly 50 grams of dirt each day. Consisting of 38 grams of fat, 2 grams of skin, 10 grams of sweat and a couple of grams of other secretions.'[5]

Some details are obviously needed. Humans produce sweat and other secretions, but no particular human organ exists for the secretion of dirt. The cited information was based on analyses of foreign particles found inside clothing, in other words of the particles that *stayed* on the fabric. Thus what *was* estimated was the condition of the garments and not of the persons who wore them, implying that the garment was treated as the primary and the person as the secondary master object of dirt. Any question of 'how much' dirt there is on a person's body surfaces runs the risk of being arbitrary. The skin of a healthy person always has a layer of dead epidermal cells, which will face you with the question of how much of it should be removed. If you want to scrub away everything that *can* be removed you must go on until you reach the bones. Not even bacteria can be identified as obviously alien and unwanted on the skin. When we say a skin disease is 'caused by' microbes, the implication is usually that the normal balance of microscopic life on the skin has been disturbed – a possible effect of many kinds of cause, including both bad hygiene and *exaggerated* hygiene.

If dirt is, as before, described as an alien and disturbing element, the question in this connection will be: *when* would an element on the body – skin cells, sweat, saliva and so on – count as a substance *alien* to it? There must of course be a great variety of answers. Functional requirements on human beings are less obvious than in the case of artefacts. A human being does not have a typical *use*, and speaking of 'use' in connection with human beings is sometimes deeply problematic. It is also difficult to define an ideally clean state for a human being. Consider children after days of intensive play on the beach or in the forest. Sniffing at their hair, one may get the feeling that they now have their own, *proper* smell to a much larger extent than they ever do in the city with daily baths.

My glass – someone else's glass

It is not always clear *what* is dirty when a person is dirty. You would typically feel your own dirt most strongly in the peripheries of your body, such as your hair, your teeth and your toes. Noxious substances inside the body are usually described as infectious or poisonous rather than dirty. The eyes of a living person are not described as (literally) dirty, apparently because foreign substances on the eye surface would immediately be something *worse* than just dirt. The sentence 'I am dirty' sometimes just means that my *clothes* are dirty. The statement, '(S)he is dirty', or '(S)he is a dirty person' may also mean that the *habits* or *home* of a person are dirty. It may even refer to a dirty mind, which indicates someone physically clean but morally questionable.

These variations concerning human dirt are directly connected with the status of the human body as a borderline object and with the philosophical question of whether 'I' is a referring expression.[6] The meaning of a name or an ordinary noun may in many cases be explained by pointing to the thing that the word stands for. However, there is no obvious *fixed* entity that would always act as the reference for the word 'I'. With 'I', I might mean my body (as in, '*I am* the same height as you') or some part of it ('*I* hurt *myself*', that is, some part of my body), or I may mean myself *as opposed to* my body or some part of it ('*I* wash *my* body', '*I* hurt *my* hand'). Finally, 'I' can be used with no particular reference to the body at all, as in '*I am* worried'. But not only the word 'I' but our talk of persons generally tends to switch between different methods of identifying the 'entity' we are talking about.

An object may quite literally function as the extension of a person. If you move a finger over a printed page, especially of printed matter from times before the development of offset techniques, you will feel microscopic differences between printed and blank parts of the page. But you feel it also if you run over the page with a toothpick. In this case, you *feel with* the end of the toothpick. The toothpick works as an organ of sense, an extended finger. Similarly, a blind man's stick functions as part of his body, and I imagine he would not like a stranger to run his fingers over the stick, precisely because the stick feels too much like an intimate extension of his sense organs.

Clothing may also take on this kind of intimate role. If I am not wearing anything at all I may feel completely naked – that is, vulnerable; a feeling that, on the other hand, I do *not* have when I am bathing. Being forced to wear other people's clothes also easily induces a sense of nakedness and loss of personal worth. Thus in *The Brothers Karamazov*, Dostoevsky includes a scene where Mitya Karamazov is placed under arrest. When Mitya has to strip quite naked in front of the police officers and take on a random array of someone else's clothing, this already makes him feel they are within their full rights to suspect him and to despise him.[7] Finally consider the role of the home, not only as the customary living space but also as the extension of one's body, as it were the *inorganic* body of the person – something that comes to the fore especially when one must leave one's home permanently. Elderly people who have found their way perfectly in their homes for years are often reported to be 'disoriented' soon after they move into a hospital milieu.

Human dirt is particularly pronounced in connection with objects that regularly make contact with the mucous membranes of the mouth and elsewhere on the body. We may think of drinking glasses, spoons, knives and forks, but also of underwear which, if it is someone else's, is carefully washed before wearing even if the owner may have had it on for an ever so fleeting moment. 'Someone else's glass' and 'someone else's underwear' must be washed before use, but we do not feel the same urge to wash before use if we are to sit down on someone else's chair.

To drink from the same glass as someone else is to be drawn into the borderline area that separates me from the other. I engage with an object which is at the same time an extension of the other person's body. This may be a cause of embarrassment but also – when I drink of the same glass *with* the other – of joy. Two Christians taking communion and two lovers sharing the same glass are not just *agreeing to* use the same vessel; the sharing gesture is an integral part of the intimacy that they cherish. I now cite Norbert Elias one last time:

> People who ate together in the way customary of the Middle Ages, taking meat with their fingers from the same dish, wine from the same goblet, soup from the same pot or the same plate . . . – such people stood in a different relationship to one another than we do . . . What was lacking in this *courtois* world, or at least had not been developed to the same degree, was the invisible wall of affects which now seems to rise between one human body and another, repelling and separating, the wall which is often perceptible today at the mere approach of something that has been in contact with the mouth or hands of someone else, and which manifests itself as embarrassment at the mere sight of many body functions of others, and often at their mere mention, or as a feeling of shame when one's own functions are exposed to the gaze of others, and by no means only then.[8]

Quite regardless of what we otherwise should think of the way Elias construes medieval culture, it strikes me as significant that his readers will immediately recognize *why* he would perceive the use of shared vessels the way he does. Human relationships are often constrained by symbolic walls reinforced by the sense of defilement while, conversely, intimacy defeats defilement.

Pure and defiling forms of intimacy

In intimacy, what is impure becomes pure; on the other hand, *forced* intimacy leaves us with a sense of being dirty. Both situations redefine the limit between clean and dirty or pure and defiled. One way to understand these changes is via the insight that the limits between an individual and his or her milieu are not fixed once and for all, and for this reason the limits between what 'belongs' and what does not are not so either. We might also say that intimacy creates its own conceptualization of the clean and the dirty. This is of course true of *all* practices: in order to understand how the concepts that belong to a practice are used you must understand the practice. Just as you cannot work with clay without getting your hands dirty, lovers cannot kiss without making contact with saliva.

However, this last sentence was misleading in more than just one way. Love is not *a practice* and it is not anyone's hobby or job like the potter's work would be. To be human is not a job and to love is to be human, to be *someone* to someone. In loving intimacy we explore and expand the limits of our bodies and souls. More-over, making contact with saliva in a kiss is not a regrettable side-effect to be put up with for the sake of the final result (whatever that might be). Not even the cleanest of people will feel disgusted by the saliva in their own mouths, but most of us cringe at the thought of someone else's saliva accidentally entering our mouths. Yet this reaction does not appear in the intimate situation; the reaction is not even suppressed, but rather it does not appear at all, because it simply makes no difference whether the saliva in one's mouth is one's own or that of one's lover. In the situation, no impure saliva exists.[9]

Excrement is often treated as the paragon of everything impure and disgusting. But even here the context matters. Parents changing the nappies of their babies are often not particularly disgusted – perhaps less than when they wipe their own behinds. Their reactions would surely be quite different if they were suddenly to note that someone's excrement has, for unknown reasons, been smeared on their garments or hands. The implication is certainly not that excrement is in the one case much cleaner than in the other. Any comparison would already presuppose that the things to be compared are placed on an equal footing and seen in relation to a shared set of criteria. But of course the very idea of undertaking a 'comparison' here would already indicate a kind of impersonal attitude not characteristic of intimacy between people.

In addition to this kind of pure and purifying intimacy there is *defiling* intimacy. In this form of contact, boundaries between people are not explored or dissolved but violated. Rape victims often speak of an overwhelming feeling of being unwashed. But this sense of defilement also comes into play in other cases of invasion of the personal sphere. In Jaan Kross's historical novel *The Czar's Madman* (1978), set in the Baltics during the reign of Nicholas I, the protagonist finds out that the father of his fiancée is a government agent, sent to spy on him and his friends. He now feels as if he, on arriving home, had suddenly discovered that the door is left wide open, the rooms have gone cold and the carpet is soiled all over with footprints. And so his life will remain unless he breaks the engagement:

> Time and again, even after I would have asked her about it ten times, and she would have sworn her innocence a hundred times – time and again, night and day, suspicion would descend upon me, so that no matter how carefully I'd lock my door, it would still remain open, because it would be impossible to close, and my floor would be covered by the muddy footprints left by a stranger . . . my own wife. For she would have become my wife only in order to gain access to the house through me, and would remain in the house as the government's ear and eye, with her father as [her employer].[10]

This passage reproduces many of the present themes with dirt as their focal point: the home as the extension of the person; the invasion of intimacy as defilement; iniquity (betrayal) as metaphorical dirt.

Confessions of an arse-wiper

Care for the elderly involves a form of soiling much more controversial and incomparably more difficult to grasp than the previous examples; it is presently one of the mined territories of the welfare state (or whatever is left of it). Professional healthcare implies a singular kind of systematic ambiguity where a *stranger* is expected to take care of tasks that one would normally only entrust to one's nearest family members – resulting in an odd and combustible mixture of personal intimacy and professional detachment.[11] This inherent ambiguity surfaced, for instance, in the 1990s, when the Norwegian trade union for nurses considered requiring extra pay for 'dirty work' – something that had been granted to rubbish collectors, oil platform workers and other members of 'male' occupations – but in the internal debate this strategy was turned down, citing the need of respect towards patients. For what would happen to their human worth if they were to be treated as producers of dirt and shit? That would also make the nursing profession into something else than what it is really about.[12] The idea that a nurse who cares for patients makes contact with dirt – just like a car mechanic would – somehow appears unacceptable, perhaps especially if you think of yourself as a future patient. And yet it is known to professionals that a very large part of the active work goes into cleaning and organizing the various bodily discharges of the patients, leaving little time to cater for psychosocial needs that may be less easily definable.[13]

This general predicament was the background of a controversial article by Jochen Temsch, published in a large German newspaper in 1994. The piece got an entire page in *Die Zeit* and invited an animated debate. Temsch, then a conscientious objector of 23 years, reported his experience of working for the public home-care service in a large West German city, visiting the homes of senior citizens for household chores and nursing work. The young man presented himself as an arse-wiper (*Arschwischer*) who does his job at the extreme ends of human orifices – 'in the place where the individual no longer exists, where he slowly disintegrates into a bad-smelling heap of wrinkled flesh'.[14] The writer's focus, how-ever, was very much on himself, *his* reactions, *his* disgust at his patients, or we might say: at his victims. Consider his visit to an old blind man who wears a colostomy pouch on a stoma (artificial anus) after surgery for colon cancer. A transparent plastic bag, with yel-lowish brown stuff inside, hangs outside the man's stomach. The blind man presses his belly to release more substance into the bag, then takes it off and gives it to Temsch for disposal. Temsch is seized by panic, and as soon as he comes home he makes his escape to the shower:

The smell sticks to every fibre of my clothing, it has fastened on my hair and it adheres to my skin. At home, I undress already in the porch; I throw the rags to the machine and go right away to the shower. I let the water run on me for hours ... But it is all no use. The smell hangs on steadily in my nose. It comes creeping from my memory, which I cannot take to a shower. Yes – there is memory for smells too.[15]

Among the numerous contributions to the ensuing debate there was one that, according to my opinion, stands out as one of the best things I have seen published on healthcare ethics. Gertrud Rückert, then 78 years old, protested against the author's 'almost autistic' fascination with his own reactions, not only as a search for cheap thrills but also as the expression of a closed mind.

The drama of the scene with a blind old man wanting to shock [Temsch] with his stoma completely escapes him: 'Look here, my boy,' the old man silently cries out, 'you are disgusted of me already after this one time, and I must carry this thing on me day and night; don't you think I am just as sick of it as you are. And now you react like all the others. It's not the bag that disgusts you. In your eyes I'm the bag.'[16]

Rückert, too, once nursed a family member who for years had to make do with a colostomy bag but, in contrast with Temsch, she does not wish to paint her experience as depressing. The problem, however, is that Temsch has only known his patients as 'heaps of misery' making one demand after the other on an already over-worked staff. Unlike Rückert, he has no experience of them as friends, family members, lovers and beloved:

> I on the other hand have known my close ones also in other ways . . . I had experience of them still in their need as partners in discussion, we have talked of our past life and the meaning of it, our faith and our hopes, and every now and then of my small everyday problems, I have touched them and I have caressed them again and again, I have held their hands and they have held mine, we have laughed a lot together.[17]

As Rückert and Temsch show us, human physical frailty is a challenge to those in the vicinity, but it is a challenge that does not admit of only *one* answer. The need to rely on strangers for help may be degrading and humiliating for those in need and equally for those whose task it is to help. But precisely the most serious case – that of following the other to the final limit of life – may also be something that tears down the walls between us, our souls and bodies.

If home-care service is seen as a whole – starting with daily help with groceries and going for walks and continuing with personal hygiene, and all this over a period of time – we have stuff for a less dramatic description. Even personal hygiene is part of life, where one thing leads to another and nothing is done without something else first having been done. Exclusively to focus on intimate hygiene is, already in advance, to make the human being into a mere producer of bodily waste, which would in fact be equally true and equally degrading if applied to completely healthy people who of course wipe themselves after using the bathroom. Rückert points out that if Temsch is shocked by the foul breath of his patients he has apparently never made acquaintance with himself in the morning. Paradoxically, he might have found the situation easier to bear if he had been able *truly* to think of his work as a mere cleaning job. Now, instead, disgust becomes for Temsch a method of shielding himself, of avoiding sympathetic involvement; quite naturally inviting the idea of a merciful end to suffering – as with an animal put out of its misery. In a similar vein, Rückert reminds us, the Australian philosopher Peter Singer has wanted to work out proper criteria for when human life should (still) be regarded as worth living. Lethal injections for the terminally ill are always just one step away if we close our minds to whatever meaning might be found even in suffering. Rückert, on the other hand, shows an attitude of openness, the insight that we can never judge things in advance. Life has something to teach us even at the onset of death, 'when, after all the insecurity, with every defence torn down, peace enters, the deeply felt acquiescence with fate, the helpless and sometimes unself-conscious surrender to the overwhelming event we call death':

On the whole the perspective of the dying is a surprisingly distanced one; it looks at life from the above. There is much to smile at in the things that we who are left behind take so very seriously.[18]

The implicit lesson of Rückert's descriptions is that utilitarianism in its pure form amounts to a kind of blindness. It is not only that the suffering that belongs to illness and death may be weighed up by positive experiences – which would be quite compatible with a utilitarian outlook – but the utilitarian focus on the simple contrast between pleasure and pain distorts experience. The present state of healthcare ethics is intelligible if we recognize that public debate on these issues has largely insulated itself against important sources of meaning. In this situation, the continuing prevalence of utilitarian arguments marks a form of entrenchment, humanly speaking all too natural given the overwhelming challenges that public healthcare is facing. And finally, the longer we live this life of tunnel vision the more will it really become the new *authentic* representation of our wish to shut out suffering and vulnerability. The question of whether a life is worth living really does look like a maths exercise in a society where you can live to be thirty without ever sitting at the bedside of someone dying; without ever holding a newborn baby in your arms.

The dead body has no value at all in terms of utility, most probably possessing negative or no more than marginally positive value. It may indeed be seen as the ultimate paradigm of pointlessness, the sad result of years of suffering and then the end – unheroic, distasteful; which is why for Kristeva 'the corpse, seen without God and outside of science, is the utmost of abjection'.[19] This idea – which, incidentally, shows that utilitarians and Kristeva have some common ground – contrasts with a more traditional view where caring for the dead body is an extension of the love and friendship that existed in the lifetime of the deceased. The body is washed, which indicates that a human corpse *may* be clean. In her essay on the tradition of washing the dead in the Swedish-speaking regions of Finland, Ulrika Wolf-Knuts describes the experience as 'thoroughly positive':[20]

Washing the corpse may also be seen as an act of love or an aesthetic measure so that family members may see a tidy body lying in state . . . An informant compares death with travel: just as you must wash before you go somewhere, to wash a deceased was a natural thing to do.[21]

Dirt as domination

Dirt may be used purposefully to break down human beings, physically as well as spiritually. Conversely, gestures at cleanliness sometimes are a way to resist the erasing of one's humanity. Both of these elements are visible in Primo Levi's memoirs from Auschwitz. Levi describes how every kind of hygiene was quite consciously made impossible from the outset, even though there were so-called washrooms and conspicuous posters with exhortations to cleanliness. When Levi was later assigned to indoors work in a chemical laboratory, his unkempt exterior could but give him the feeling that no form of human community was imaginable between him and his civilian co-workers from the outside. What with the conditions of the camp, Levi could at first not understand why his fellow inmate, Steinlauf, demonstratively undertook a daily simulated morning bath, scrubbing himself energetically but with little result over the sink with filthy water and without soap. For the sake of whom or what would he do it? Gradually the logic of it dawned on him,

> that precisely because the Lager was a great machine to reduce us to beasts, we must not become beasts; that even in this place one can survive, and therefore one must want to survive, to tell the story, to bear witness; and that to survive we must force ourselves to save at least the skeleton, the scaffolding, the form of civilization. We are slaves, deprived of every right, exposed to every insult, condemned to certain death, but we still possess one power, and we must defend it with all our strength for it is the last – the power to refuse our consent. So we must certainly wash

our faces without soap in dirty water and dry ourselves on our jackets. We must polish our shoes, not because the regulation states it, but for dignity and propriety. We must walk erect, without dragging our feet, not in homage to Prussian discipline but to remain alive, not to begin to die.[22]

Auschwitz inmates were left with practically nothing. Yet by continuing the daily routine of washing they might try at least to preserve the *memory* of a normal life, which not only unmasked the mockery of Lager regulations but also might give them the determination to survive.

In his short novel *One Day in the Life of Ivan Denisovich* (1962), Alexander Solzhenitsyn depicts several scenes that focus on cleanliness in extreme circumstances. Despite the primitive conditions of the Gulag, the inmates uphold a kind of notional cleanliness embodied in a number of implicit rules and split-second considerations. You would deliberate whether to let someone else use your cigarette holder; you would lick and wipe clean your personal spoon (which is never washed) on your jacket, but you would not lick other people's soup-plates. At meals, it would be uncouth to spit fish-bones directly on the floor, but bones are left on heaps on the table – from where the next group will certainly sweep them all down. Leftovers do end up on the floor, but even this is a case of propriety and human self-respect: the incoming group would of course, just like the previous one, want to eat from a *clean* table. In such ways the inmates would follow their own set of rules to create a standard of cleanliness relative to the circumstances.

In some situations, the precarious feeling of being clean in a world of dirt would, however, be badly undermined. Ivan Denisovich is overcome by the sense of being unclean at the moment when, having contracted a fever, he enters the (relatively) clean milieu of the dispensary. Like Levi in the laboratory at Auschwitz, Ivan is struck by the contrast between his dishevelled appearance and 'that spick-and-span room'. He takes off his cap as before an authority and sits down uncomfortably at the very end of a bench by the wall, 'involuntarily emphasizing that he was unfamiliar with the place and that he'd come there on some minor matter' – as if preparing to take to flight either from himself or from the obviously 'clean' medical staff.[23]

Purity and unworldly life

The mutual dependence between dirt, responsibility and personal identity is the starting point of the well-known symbolic association between physical cleanliness and moral purity. Cleanliness is culture, responsible behaviour and honesty, but it may also mark dull and shallow thinking with an exclusive focus on the material world to the detriment of spiritual values. Conversely, lack of cleanliness may be seen as barbaric, but when it turns into a form of ascetic practice, the ascetic puts a distance between herself and every worldly concern, including personal hygiene; the 'holy fools' of pre-revolutionary Russia would be an example of this.[24]

It is possible that this form of ascetic practice can be historically traced back to neo-Platonist ideas about freeing oneself of the body (even though Plotinus, the greatest of the neo-Platonists, *did* wash himself; the usual, opposite opinion goes back to Porphyry's biography, where he simply says his beloved teacher avoided *public* baths).[25] In this connection we should once more think of the Latin *sordidus, sordere*. In ancient Rome, these expressions referred to the practice of wearing unwashed garments, not shaving and generally assuming an unkempt appearance as a sign of mourning. The death of a family member or, for instance, facing accusations of some serious wrongdoing, would be events that place you in a state of exception. Conversely, *purus* ('pure') was used for a person who had finished mourning or who had cleared his reputation in a court of law.

The neglect of cleanliness as an ascetic practice is based on the idea that you should focus your cares on your inner or spiritual life, not on externalities. Thus, in conscious opposition to rabbinic law, Christ declared that man does not become impure by eating with unwashed hands. Whatever goes in through the mouth will come out naturally in due course, but what comes out through the mouth can be defiling – namely for those who speak lies and evil.[26] The logic of this kind of spiritual purity trumps the demands of everyday cleanliness, robbing them of any validity they may have had.

The early part of Genesis, which may be treated as a representation of the world view of Christian civilization, includes some intriguing expressions of our ambiguous attitude towards material culture. God, the Supreme Architect, gives man and woman the Garden of Eden 'to till it and to keep it'; he tells them to multiply and fill the earth.[27] And yet every means available for the tasks appears questionable. Knowledge of good and evil is a forbidden fruit; work and childbirth are imposed on humanity as punishments. Other parts of the Old Testament extol the values of justice, industry and family, as when God promises that Abraham will be the father of a large people.[28] But the impression remains that underneath, human history as a whole is a rather dubious thing. Cultural historian Egon Friedell notes this ambiguity and writes in reaction to it:

> Through the rolling, thundering waves of millennia there sounds a voice of comfort and warning: Man's kingdom is not of this world. But beside it comes a roaring second voice: This world, full of splendour and shadow is yours, it belongs to human beings; it is your work and you are its work; you cannot escape it. And even if you could, you should not! The way it is created, terrible and wonderful, you must be true to it. This unresolved dissonance is the theme of world history.[29]

Wittgenstein writes in his *Notebooks*: 'The usual way of looking at things sees objects as it were from the midst of them.' But, as he continues, to see them from the perspective of eternity, '*sub specie aeternitatis*', is to see them 'from outside. In such a way that they have the whole world as background.'[30] Formulating the contrast in this way also throws some light on my aims with the present book, for the idea was precisely to look at things and practices 'from the midst of them' – or perhaps better, to find out *what it is* to look at things and practices from the midst of them; for even that is a question to be taken seriously.

REFERENCES

Preface

1 Oswald Spengler, *Der Mensch und die Technik* (Munich, 1931), pp. 28–9, emphasis in the original.
2 For a discussion of approaches to dirt in social theory, see Carol Wolkowitz, 'Linguistic Leakiness or Really Dirty? Dirt in Social Theory', in *Dirt: New Geographies of Cleanliness and Contamination*, ed. Ben Campkin and Rosie Cox (London, 2007); Rosie Cox, 'Introduction', ibid.

PART I:
THE PHILOSOPHICAL LANDSCAPE OF 'DIRTY' AND 'CLEAN'

1 Friedrich Nietzsche, *Der Wille zur Macht*, in Friedrich Nietzsche, *Werke*, Band XVI (Leipzig, 1911), §556, pp. 60–61, my translation.

1 Dirt in Philosophy and Culture

1 Ludwig Wittgenstein, *Philosophical Investigations*, ed. G.E.M. Anscombe and G. H. von Wright, trans. G.E.M. Anscombe (Oxford, 1953), I:§122.
2 Compare Huizinga's concept of *Homo ludens,* the playing and joking man; see Johan Huizinga, *Homo ludens. Versuch einer Bestimmung des Spielelements der Kultur* (Amsterdam, 1994).
3 Giambattista Vico, *Scienza Nuova*, §332–3. The quotes from Vico and Eliot are included in Peter Winch, 'Understanding a Primitive Society', in Peter Winch, *Ethics and Action* (London, 1972), pp. 8–49, at pp. 44, 47.
4 My starting point is, in other words, that the normal, *natural* human habitat is a *cultural* environment. Insofar as we want to apply the term 'natural' at all to humans, the unchecked war of every man against every man – the war that Thomas Hobbes dignified with the term 'state of nature'

– must instead be described as unnatural. Where such a state prevails, a
background of civil wars or other past disasters inevitably shines through.

5 Cf. Ludwig Wittgenstein, *On Certainty* (New York, 1972), §§96–9.

6 Ludwig Wittgenstein, *Philosophical Investigations*, I:§129.

7 R. G. Collingwood, 'Preliminary Discussion: The Idea of a Philosophy
of Something, and, in Particular, a Philosophy of History (1927)', in R. G.
Collingwood, *The Idea of History: With Lectures, 1926–1928*, revd edn,
ed. Jan van der Dussen (Oxford, 2005), pp. 335–58, at p. 351.

8 Collingwood calls concepts which are 'applicable to everything that exists',
'transcendentals' (Collingwood, 'The Idea of a Philosophy of Something',
pp. 351–2). The concept of teacup is 'applicable only to a certain class of
things but not to others' (p. 352).

9 François Dagognet, *Rematérialiser. Matières et matérialismes* (Paris, 1985).

10 Recent controversies around various 'Mohammed caricatures' seem,
moreover, directly to link art wars with 'the war on terrorism'. The
cartoonist's stated goal has in many cases been precisely to cause offence
– as opposed to Serrano's work, which expresses a recognizable idea of
theological relevance and thus, unlike a work that *only* aims to cause
offence, clearly falls under freedom of expression.

11 Andrew Hudgins, 'Piss Christ – Andres Serrano 1987', *Slate*, 19 April
2000, www.slate.com/articles/arts/poem/2000/04, accessed 1 June 2014.
Porphyry wrote, in his *Against the Christians*: 'How can we admit that
the divine became an embryo, and that after its birth, it was wrapped up
in swaddling clothes, covered with blood, bile, and even worse things?'
Porphyry, *Against the Christians*, frag. 77, quoted in Pierre Hadot, *Plotinus
or the Simplicity of Vision* (Chicago, IL, 1998), p. 23. Cf. Plato, *The Republic*,
in *The Dialogues of Plato*, trans. Benjamin Jowett (Chicago, IL, 1952),
pp. 295–441, at p. 381b–c.

12 Nina Björkman, 'Gränsfallsbilder', *Hufvudstadsbladet*, 13 April 2002, p. 14,
my translation.

13 For example, the exhibition 'Dirt: The Filthy Reality of Everyday Life'
at the Wellcome Collection, London, 24 March–31 August 2011, was
accompanied by interdisciplinary symposia and an edited collection, *Dirt:
The Filthy Reality of Everyday Life*, ed. Nadine Monem (London, 2011).

14 André Comte-Sponville, *A Small Treatise on the Great Virtues: The Uses
of Philosophy in Everyday Life* (New York, 2003), p. 174 (the author fails to
mention that whatever lives also kills).

15 See for instance Julia Kristeva, *Powers of Horror: An Essay on Abjection*
(New York, 1982), p. 210.

16 Zygmunt Bauman, *Postmodernity and Its Discontents* (Cambridge, 1997);
Martha C. Nussbaum, '"Secret Sewers of Vice": Disgust, Bodies, and the
Law', in *The Passions of Law*, ed. Susan Bandes (New York, 1999),
pp. 19–62; Klaus Theweleit, *Male Fantasies*, vol. I, trans. Stephen Conway
(Cambridge, 1987); also see Comte-Sponville, *Small Treatise*, pp. 174–5.
Bauman's book title *Postmodernity and Its Discontents* is obviously an
allusion to Freud's *Civilization and Its Discontents*.

17 Nussbaum, 'Secret Sewers of Vice'.

18 As examples of how disgust is expressed in everyday life, Nussbaum
mentions the fact that 'we wash our bodies . . . cleanse ourselves of
offending odours with toothbrush and mouthwash, sniff our armpits
when nobody is looking' (ibid., p. 20) as well as 'the ability to wash and to
dispose of wastes' (p. 24). She connects 'focus on cleanliness' with disgust
(p. 31).

19 Colin McGinn advances, much like Nussbaum, the claim that disgust
is our way to symbolically suppress the insight of our mortality. Colin
McGinn, *The Meaning of Disgust* (Oxford, 2011). For a review, see Nina
Strohminger, 'The Meaning of Disgust: A Refutation', *Emotion Review*, VI/3
(2014), pp. 214–16.

20 William Ian Miller, *The Anatomy of Disgust* (Cambridge, MA, 1997); Paul
Rozin and April E. Fallon, 'A Perspective on Disgust', *Psychological Review*
XCIV (1987), pp. 23–41.

21 Nussbaum, 'Secret Sewers of Vice', p. 23.

22 Ibid., pp. 23–4.

23 Ibid., p. 25.

24 Ibid.

25 Ibid., p. 33. But doesn't this indicate that Nussbaum partly agrees with – or
at least does not want to quarrel with – the basic misogynistic idea that
women, more than men, are to be viewed through the lens of their bodies
and sexuality?

26 Ibid., p. 23.

27 Ibid., p. 24. Nussbaum is quoting Rozier's research.

28 Nussbaum admits that 'decayed and moldy' (ibid.) vegetarian
substances may also be disgusting, as well as vegetarian substances
that remind us of animal products. If Sartre had been around for Rozin's
laboratory test he might have told him about his feelings about treacle,
a thoroughly vegetarian product. Nussbaum also points out that tears,
unlike other human body fluids, are not perceived as dirty. According
to her this is because weeping is considered an exclusively human

activity. She does not consider the other obvious explanation, the fact that tears, unlike mucus, blood and urine, do not leave marks on clothing and furniture.

29 In trying to compose a list of typically disgusting objects, it would be natural to focus on the relation between the disgusting/distasteful and the *edible* in general. Biologically and ethologically, it is hardly a coincidence that there is often just a small step from the delicious to the disgusting: amplified reactions of disgust protect us above all from harmful substances that we might otherwise consider eating.

30 Nussbaum distinguishes between disgust and the sensory reaction of distaste. The existence of instinctive reactions against, for instance, the ingestion of faecal matter does then not imply that dung is always an object of disgust – for instance, when it is used as fertilizer or fuel.

31 Ludwig Wittgenstein, *Blue and Brown Books* (New York, 1965), p. 18.

32 Per Svensson, *Svenska hem. En bok om hur vi bor och varför* (Stockholm, 2002), p. 90.

33 Colin Blackstock, 'Cleaner Cleans Up Hirst's Ashtray Art', *The Guardian*, 19 October 2001, available at www.theguardian.com.

34 In this sense, philosophy must be 'a working on oneself . . . On one's way of seeing things. (And what one expects of them.)' Ludwig Wittgenstein, *Culture and Value*, ed. G. H. von Wright and Heikki Nyman, trans. Peter Winch (Chicago, IL, 1984), p. 16e.

2 A Brief History of Dirt in Philosophy

1 In analogy with Huizinga's *sub specie ludi* – from the point of view of play.

2 Cf. Peter Winch, *The Idea of a Social Science and Its Relation to Philosophy* (London, 1958), p. 9.

3 Heraclitus, Fragment B5, quoted in translation by Osborne in Catherine Osborne, 'Heraclitus', in *Routledge History of Philosophy*, vol. I: *From the Beginning to Plato*, ed. C.C.W. Taylor (London, 1997), pp. 88–127, at pp. 90–91.

4 *Egyptian Book of the Dead*, ed. E. A. Wallis Budge (New York, 1967), p. 258, brackets mine.

5 Ibid., p. 289, brackets in the original.

6 Heraclitus, 'Fragments of Heraclitus', trans. John Burnet (1912), available at https://en.wikisource.org/wiki, Fragment 37, accessed 16 October 2015.

7 Ibid., 61.

8 Ibid., 13.

9 Osborne, 'Heraclitus', p. 93.

10 Ibid., p. 90, and endnote 11, p. 118. An alternative translation of Fragment 5 by Burnet runs: 'They vainly purify themselves by defiling themselves with blood, just as if one who had stepped into the mud were to wash his feet in mud. And they pray to these images, as if one were to talk with a man's house, knowing not what gods or heroes are.' Heraclitus, 'Fragments', 5.

11 Fragment 78, quoted in translation by Osborne in Osborne, 'Heraclitus', p. 93.

12 Heraclitus, 'Fragments', 70.

13 Ibid., 96.

14 [Heraclitus], *Heraklit, Fragmente*, Greek and German, ed. Bruno Snell (Munich, 1926), Fragment B124, my translation.

15 Heraclitus, 'Fragments', 69.

16 Ibid., 102.

17 Martin Heidegger, *Being and Time*, trans. John Macquarrie and Edward Robinson (Oxford, 2001), pp. [68] 96–7.

18 Plato, *Parmenides*, in *The Dialogues of Plato*, trans. Benjamin Jowett (Chicago, IL, 1952), pp. 486–511, at 130d.

19 Plato, *The Sophist*, in *The Dialogues of Plato*, trans. Benjamin Jowett (Chicago, IL, 1952), pp. 551–79, at 257d–258a; Plato, *The Republic*, ibid., pp. 295–441, at 476a. However, the cited passage in *The Republic* is not so much a discussion as a mention of the Theory of Forms. Moreover, the conclusions in *The Sophist* are not presented in the name of Socrates, Plato's usual mouthpiece, but of 'an Eleatic stranger'.

20 I am grateful to Prof. Nicholas White for information on the debate; personal communication, 18 August 2003.

21 Plato, *Parmenides*, 130e.

22 Aristotle, *Problems*, Books I–XXI, trans. W. S. Hett (London, 1961), at Book XIII, pp. 306–15. The *Problems* belongs to the post-Aristotelian tradition of the third century BCE. All in all it is a work of 36 books summing up the then available knowledge from botany, zoology and medicine all the way to music. The main part is traceable to authentic Aristotelian notes taken by members of the Peripatos.

23 Aristotle, *Problems*, 907b, 909a, 908b.

24 Aristotle, *Generation of Animals*, trans. A. L. Peck (Cambridge, MA, 1946), Book IV, 769b–773a.

25 Hesiod, 'Works and Days', in *Hesiod and Theognis*, trans. and intro. D. Wender (Harmondsworth, 1986), pp. 59–86, at v. 105–202.

26 Ibid., v. 173.

27 The Bible, New Revised Standard Version (NRSV), www.biblestudytools.
    com, accessed 8 June 2016, Romans 8:19–23.

28 Timo Joutsivuo, 'Raamatun pitkäikäisyyden salaisuus', *Tieteessä tapahtuu*,
    7 (2003), pp. 32–4.

29 Tomas Mansikka, 'Alkemisk uppbyggelselitteratur', *Finsk Tidskrift*,
    CCLI–CCLII (2002), pp. 397–408.

30 Martin Luther, *The Table Talk of Martin Luther*, trans. and ed. William
    Hazlitt (London, 1872), at DCCV, p. 326.

31 Isaiah 1.22, 25 (NRSV).

32 Malachi 3.3 (NRSV).

33 Revelation 21, 18–21 (NRSV).

34 François Dagognet, in *Rématerialiser: Matières et materialismes* (Paris,
    1885). pp. 37–9, argues that certain tendencies in alchemy arrested the
    development of chemistry for a long time. Alchemy concentrated on
    freeing the essence or 'spirit' from its unworthy frame, which also implied
    preference for 'pure' materials and forms such as white crystals instead of
    exploring the potentialities of slag products.

35 Giovanni Pico della Mirandola, *Oration on the Dignity of Man* (Chicago,
    IL, 1956).

36 Ibid., p. 16.

37 Ibid., p. 18.

38 Ibid., p. 49.

39 Ibid., p. 51.

40 Ibid., p. 55.

41 Galileo Galilei, *Sagiattore*; quoted from Oswald Spengler, *Der Untergang
    des Abendlades*, Band I (Munich, 1921), p. 10.

42 John Locke, *An Essay Concerning Human Understanding* (London, 1867),
    at Book II, Ch. VIII, §§15, 14. See also §22: 'The bulk, figure, number,
    situation, and motion or rest of their solid parts; those are in them
    [the objects], whether we perceive them or no.'

43 Ibid., Book II, Ch. VIII, §14.

44 Ibid., §17.

45 On secondary qualities in general, including a historical account
    of the development of the idea, see P.M.S. Hacker, *Appearance and
    Reality: An Investigation into Perception and Perceptual Qualities*
    (Oxford, 1991).

46 Locke presents different lists in different passages of his work (all included
    in Locke, *Essay*, Book II, Ch. VIII): 'bulk, figure and motion of parts' (§17);
    'size, figure, number, and motion of its parts' (§18); 'bulk, figure, number,

situation, and motion or rest of their solid parts' (§23); 'bulk, figure, texture, or motion' (§24).

47 Locke, however, introduces a tripartite division of another kind where the 'third' kind of quality in bodies is their power to effect changes in other bodies, as when the sun has the power to melt wax. Ibid., Book II, Ch. VIII, §§23–4.

48 Jonas Frykman, 'Hel och ren. Kropp och tanke hos bönder och borgare', in *Den kultiverade människan*, ed. J. Frykman and O. Löfgren (Lund, 1979), pp. 131–220, at p. 135.

3 Dirty and Clean: Main Distinctions

1 Aristotle, *Politics*, trans. Benjamin Jowett (Oxford, 1938), I.5, 1254a.

2 *The Concise Oxford Dictionary of Current English*, ed. H. W. Fowler and F. G. Fowler (Oxford, 1956), p. 339.

3 Also see Jerzy Faryno, 'Neskol'ko obščih soobraženij po povodu konceptov "grjaznyj/čistyj"', *Studia Litteraria Polono-Slavica*, IV (1999), pp. 59–62.

4 Compare Nussbaum's idea of making a survey of 'all disgust objects' (see Martha C. Nussbaum, '"Secret Sewers of Vice": Disgust, Bodies, and the Law', in *The Passions of Law*, ed. Susan Bandes (New York, 1999), p. 24, and Chapter One of the present volume). On the other hand, coal dust may be called 'a dirty substance' (as pointed out to me by Ieuan Lloyd, in discussion, 15 April 1995). Coal dust is dirty roughly in the same sense as water is wet: we must think of coal dust in *contact* with some other substance, such as the hands and clothes of those who work with it. The point would be that contact with coal dust unfailingly creates the need of cleaning.

5 Also see Christian Enzensberger, *Grösserer Versuch über den Schmutz* (Munich, 1970), p. 30.

6 *Dirt: The Filthy Reality of Everyday Life*, ed. Nadine Mone (London, 2011), p. 67.

7 According to *Wikipedia*, Croak's dirt sculpture starts with sculpting with clay and using the statue to create a set of moulds. Afterwards, 'Croak digs up or acquires a large amount of dirt and dries it with the aid of large fans. [Next], Croak mixes the dirt with a binder, then pours the mixture into the mould. [Finally], once set, the pieces of the sculpture are then reassembled and glued together with the same dirt and binder mixture with which they were created.' *Wikipedia*, 'James Croak', https://en.wikipedia.org, accessed 13 June 2016.

8   Jean-Paul Sartre, *Being and Nothingness: An Essay on Phenomenological Ontology* (London, 1969), pp. 610–12.

9   Thomas Leddy, 'Everyday Surface Aesthetic Qualities: "Neat", "Messy", "Clean", "Dirty"', *Journal of Aesthetics and Art Criticism*, LIII (1995), pp. 259–68. The essay is included with revisions in Thomas Leddy, *The Extraordinary in the Ordinary: The Aesthetics of Everyday Life* (Peterborough, ON, 2012).

10 See for example Georges Bataille, 'La valeur d'usage de D.A.F. de Sade', in Georges Bataille, *Oeuvres complètes*, vol. II (Paris, 1970), pp. 54–73; Mary Douglas, *Purity and Danger: An Analysis of Concepts of Pollution and Taboo* (Harmondsworth, 1970); Julia Kristeva, *Powers of Horror: An Essay on Abjection* (New York, 1982); Nussbaum, 'Secret Sewers of Vice'.

11 Leddy, 'Everyday Surface Aesthetic Qualities', p. 262.

12 Ibid.

13 Le Corbusier [Charles-Edouard Jeanneret], *L'Art décoratif d'aujourd'hui*, *1925* (Paris, 2008), p. 191, italics in the original, my translation. Le Corbusier argued, 'If a house is all white, the design of things shows itself without any possible transgression . . . Whitewash is absolute, everything shows itself, everything is outlined absolutely, black on *white*; it is honest and loyal . . . It is the eye of truth. Whitewash is extremely moral.' Ibid., p. 193, italics in the original, my translation.

14 Ibid., p. 260.

15 Aristotle, *Metaphysics*, trans. W. D. Ross, in *The Works of Aristotle*, ed. W. D. Ross, vol. VIII (Oxford, 1960), pp. 1023b–1024a.

16 Cf. Faryno, 'Neskol'ko obščih soobraženij', p. 60, my translation: 'The already empty plate at the unfinished dinner, with the guest still holding on to his knife and fork, is still "clean"; while the same plate at the same dinner, but with the guest waiting for the next course, is already "dirty".'

17 André Comte-Sponville, *A Small Treatise on the Great Virtues: The Uses of Philosophy in Everyday Life* (New York, 2003), pp. 174–5.

18 Ibid., p. 182.

19 Faryno, 'Neskol'ko obščih soobraženij'. On the other hand, the idea of 'ethnic cleansing' associates with the contrast of dirty vs clean. The ethnically alien population is not defined as impure on the account of mixing with another group, but the (unmixed) ethnic group as a whole counts as dirt on the body of the nation.

20 Karl Marx notes that it is in the 'spirit' of the English language 'to use a Teutonic word for the actual thing, and a Romance word for its reflexion'.

Karl Marx, *Capital*, vol. I, trans. Samuel Moore and Edward Aveling (New York, 1967), p. 36, fn. 1.

21 Leddy, 'Everyday Surface Aesthetic Qualities', p. 264.

22 Lars Hertzberg, in discussion (no date).

23 A.D.M. Walker, 'The Ideal of Sincerity', *Mind*, LXXXVII, New Series (1978), pp. 481–97, at p. 490.

24 Ibid.

25 Ibid., p. 491.

26 Douglas, *Purity and Danger*, p. 12.

27 Anna Magdalena L. Midtgaard, 'The Dust of History and the Politics of Preservation', paper for the Nordic Summer University Winter Symposium, Circle 4: Information, Technology, Aesthetics, 3–5 March 2006, Helsinki.

28 Barbara Lönnqvist, email to the author, 15 March 1997, and discussion (no date).

29 Peter Winch, *The Idea of a Social Science and Its Relation to Philosophy* (London, 1958).

30 Lars Hertzberg, discussion (no date).

31 On the relation between 'brute facts' and evaluative descriptions, see G.E.M. Anscombe, 'On Brute Facts', in G.E.M. Anscombe, *Collected Philosophical Papers*, vol. III (Minneapolis, MN, 1981), pp. 22–5.

32 Thus, according to Nora Hämäläinen, our understanding of facts includes or points towards a hierarchy of value; a 'dynamic principle of our lived, everyday experience', which 'is not of our own making, and which places demands on us'. Nora Hämäläinen, 'What is a Wittgensteinian Neo-Platonist?: Iris Murdoch, Metaphysics and Metaphor', *Philosophical Papers*, XLIII/2 (2014), pp. 191–225, at pp. 217, 215.

4 Reductionism and the Role of Science

1 E. J. Lowe, 'How are Ordinary Objects Possible?', *The Monist*, LXXXVIII/4 (2005), pp. 510–33.

2 John Heil, 'Real Tables', *The Monist*, LXXXVIII/4 (2005), pp. 493–509, at p. 497.

3 Lowe, 'How are Ordinary Objects Possible?', p. 511.

4 A. S. Eddington, *The Nature of the Physical World* (New York, 1929), pp. ix, ix–x, quoted in Heil, 'Real Tables', p. 498. Wittgenstein addresses a similar case, possibly thinking of Eddington: 'We have been told by popular scientists that the floor on which we stand is not solid, as it

appears to common sense, as it has been discovered that the wood consists of particles filling space so thinly that it can almost be called empty.' Ludwig Wittgenstein, *Blue and Brown Books* (New York, 1965), p. 45. He continues (pp. 45–6): 'in this example the word "solidity" was used wrongly and it seemed that we had shown that nothing really was solid'. I should also point out that Heil takes Eddington to task for lack of clarity about his final position. The right position is not that nothing is solid but that 'physics has provided us with a deeper understanding of the nature of substantiality' (Heil, 'Real Tables', p. 503).

5   Eddington, *The Nature of the Physical World*, p. xii, quoted in Heil, 'Real Tables', p. 498.

6   Heil, 'Real Tables', p. 497.

7   In writing these paragraphs, I have profited from discussion with Martin Gustafsson, Camilla Kronqvist and Hugo Strandberg at the Philosophy Research Seminar, Åbo Akademi University, 8 April 2015.

8   Lynne Rudder Baker, 'A Metaphysics of Ordinary Things and Why We Need It', *Philosophy*, LXXXIII (2008), pp. 5–24, at pp. 23–4.

9   By-products and slag are not impurities in the usual sense. They have a well-defined role in the industrial chemical process but in the end they are separated from the final product. In relation to the latter they count as impurities but they do not necessarily indicate impurity or pollution in the raw material. A slag product can later be turned into the raw material of some other process. This was the case with coal-tar, which was a by-product from the production of gas. The nineteenth century saw the explosive development of aniline pigments based on coal-tar. The external look of modern culture is to a large extent a product of the aniline revolution. Its most immediately visible consequence was the increased use of blue pigments which up to that point had been particularly expensive. For more on the aniline revolution, see François Dagognet, *Rématerialiser. Matières et materialismes* (Paris, 1885), p. 36.

10 Socialstyrelsens nämnd för hälsoupplysning, *Personlig hygien*, 1977. Stockholm: Committee on Health Education, National Swedish Board of Health and Welfare. Quoted and translated from Gudrun Linn, 'Ur "Badrum och städning"', *Res Publica*, LVII (2002), pp. 21–9, at pp. 26, 28.

11 Norbert Elias, *The Civilizing Process*, vol. I: *The History of Manners*, trans. Edmund Jephcott (Oxford, 1978), pp. 158–9, 115–16, 135, and in particular, note 124 (pp. 305–7).

12 Elias, *The Civilizing Process*, vol. I, pp. 158–9. Also see pp. 107, 115, 126–7.

13 For instance, Strohminger points to some important biological functions of the feelings of disgust. However, it must be kept in mind that 'dirty' and 'disgusting' are not synonymous. Nina Strohminger, '*The Meaning of Disgust*: A Refutation', *Emotion Review*, VI/3 (2014).

14 Martha C. Nussbaum, '"Secret Sewers of Vice": Disgust, Bodies, and the Law', in *The Passions of Law*, ed. Susan Bandes (New York, 1999), p. 25.

15 Ibid., p. 32, italics mine. Nussbaum presents her suggestion as a protest against 'Freudian psychoanalyst Norbert Elias' who, she believes, 'argues that the more things a society recognizes as disgusting, the more advanced it is in civilization' and that 'the more we focus on cleanliness and the more intolerant we become of slime, filth, and our own bodily products, the more civilized we are' (p. 31). Nussbaum finds this 'utterly unconvincing'. The problem with Nussbaum's rejection of Elias is that she ignores the distinction between *culture* and *civilization*, which was a central idea for Elias and generally the German debate at the time he wrote. Unlike Nussbaum, Elias thinks of the advance of 'civilization' descriptively as the transition from one form of social organization to another, not as *moral* progress. 'It is necessary', he writes, 'at least while considering this process, to attempt to suspend all the feelings of embarrassment and superiority, all the value judgements and criticism associated with the concepts "civilization" or "uncivilized" . . . In reality, our terms "civilized" and "uncivilized" do not constitute an antithesis of the kind that exists between "good" and "bad", but represent stages in a development which, moreover, is still continuing' (Elias, *The Civilizing Process*, vol. I, p. 59).

16 Aldous Huxley, *Brave New World* [1932], www.idph.com, accessed 13 October 2015, Ch. 3, pp. 27–8.

17 Sigmund Freud, *Totem and Taboo*, authorized trans. by A. A. Brill (New York, 1946), pp. 85–6, italics mine.

PART II: 'DIRTY' AND 'FORBIDDEN': ANTHROPOLOGICAL REDUCTIONISM AND ITS LIMITS

1 Ludwig Wittgenstein, 'Remarks on Frazer's *Golden Bough*', in Ludwig Wittgenstein, *Philosophical Occasions, 1912–1951*, ed. James Klagge and Alfred Nordmann (Indianapolis, IN, 1993), pp. 115–55, at p. 119.

5 Ritual, Disorder and Pollution

1 Mary Douglas, *Purity and Danger: An Analysis of Concepts of Pollution and Taboo* (Harmondsworth, 1970), p. 48.

2 Émile Durkheim, *The Elementary Forms of the Religious Life* (London, 1968), pp. 28–9, 84–5.

3 Ibid., pp. 127–33.

4 Douglas, *Purity and Danger*, p. 210.

5 For example ibid., p. 14.

6 Ibid., p. 48.

7 Ibid., p. 194.

8 Ibid., p. 190.

9 Ibid., p. 200. Sartre is explicitly discussed on pp. 51, 191.

10 Ibid., pp. 200–201.

11 Ibid., p. 193.

12 Jean-Paul Sartre, *Nausea*, trans. Lloyd Alexander (New York, 1964).

13 Douglas, *Purity and Danger*, p. 15.

14 Ibid., p. 50.

15 Ibid., Ch. 10.

16 Ibid., p. 202.

17 Cf. Zygmunt Bauman, *Postmodernity and Its Discontents* (Cambridge, 1997); Christian Enzensberger, *Grösserer Versuch über den Schmutz* (Munich, 1970); Jonas Frykman, 'Hel och ren. Kropp och tanke hos bönder och borgare', in *Den kultiverade människan*, ed. J. Frykman and O. Löfgren (Lund, 1979), pp. 131–220; Julia Kristeva, *Powers of Horror: An Essay on Abjection* (New York, 1982); Martha C. Nussbaum, '"Secret Sewers of Vice": Disgust, Bodies, and the Law', in *The Passions of Law*, ed. Susan Bandes (New York, 1999), pp. 19–62; Roger Fayet, 'Moderne Reinigung, postmoderne Kompostierung. Über ein abfalltheoretisches Modell und die eigentlichen Signaturen zweier Zeitalter', in *Verlangen nach Reinheit oder Lust auf Schmutz? Gestaltungskonzepte zwischen rein und unrein*, ed. Roger Fayet (Vienna, 2003), pp. 15–40.

18 Douglas, *Purity and Danger*, pp. 47–8.

19 Ibid., p. 191.

20 Ibid., p. 48.

21 Ibid.

22 The Swedish translation of *Purity and Danger* renders 'out of place' in the quoted passage as '*olämplig*' ('improper') and '*dirty*' as '*stötande*'

('offending'), which makes the argument as a whole less conspicuously implausible. To place one's shoes on a table is (often) offending precisely because it is improper. But this of course fails to support the thesis that dirt implies disorder. Dr Henry Nygård (personal correspondence, 18 March 2002) has notified me of the discrepancy between the translation and the original.

23 Advertising campaign, London Heathrow, 2003.

24 Douglas, *Purity and Danger*, p. 52.

25 Ibid., pp. 42–3.

26 Leviticus 11:7 (NRSV).

27 Leviticus 11:6 (NRSV).

28 Douglas, *Purity and Danger*, p. 68.

29 Ibid., pp. 69–70.

30 Ibid., pp. 70–71.

31 Leviticus 11:2–8 (NRSV), italics mine.

32 Leviticus 11:26–8 (NRSV), italics mine.

33 Leviticus 11:29–32 (NRSV), italics mine.

34 Douglas, *Purity and Danger*, p. 70, italics mine.

35 *Encyclopedia Judaica* 1971, vol. VI (Jerusalem, 1971), p. 31 ('Dietary Laws').

36 Douglas, *Purity and Danger*, pp. 70–71.

37 We may distinguish between *disorder* and *lack of order*. Disorder implies that some item fails to occupy the place assigned to it. A library arranged according to subject matter is in disorder if there are anthropology books on the cookery shelf. Lack of order, on the other hand, means the *absence* of an organizing principle. The bookshelf will lack order as long as it is not *meant* to be in a particular order, but it is not in disorder and cannot be until there is a principle of organization. Lars Hertzberg, in discussion (no date).

38 Isaiah 1:15–16, 18 (NRSV).

39 Peter Winch, *The Idea of a Social Science and Its Relation to Philosophy* (London, 1958), p. 88.

40 Douglas, *Purity and Danger*, p. 49.

41 Ibid., p. 51. Douglas refers to Sartre's description of the experience of viscosity in *Being and Nothingness* (London, 1989), pp. 610–12, originally published 1943, an account in close parallel with the story of Roquentin's experiences in 1938. One may ask, however, whether the experience would have to be nauseating. Sometimes Sartre's emphasis on the negative aspects of Roquentin's experiences has been put down to the effects of a certain 'bad trip' by Sartre.

42 Jean-Paul Sartre, 'Une idée fondamentale de la phénoménologie de Husserl: l'intentionnalité', in Jean-Paul Sartre, *La transcendance de l'ego, esquisse d'une description phénoménologique* (Paris, 1981), Appendix v, pp. 109–13, at p. 113, trans. and italics mine.

43 Douglas, *Purity and Danger*, p. 49, italics mine.

44 The probable explanation is that Douglas runs together two arguments: one about the philosophy and the other about the psychology of perception. The philosophical argument is a Kantian one: all perception presupposes order. We perceive the world as ordered in terms of time, space and causality. The argument from the psychology of perception involves the assumption that perception is conservative. We cannot easily adjust to unfamiliar surroundings and we tend to interpret those by imposing patterns derived from past experience.

45 Douglas, *Purity and Danger*, p. 190.

6 Repressing the 'Other': The Myth of Abjection

1 Immanuel Kant, *Critique of Pure Reason*, trans. Norman Kemp Smith (London, 1964), A80/B106, A70/B95.

2 Ibid., B126, B165.

3 Émile Durkheim, *The Elementary Forms of the Religious Life* (London, 1968), p. 17.

4 Cf. Julia Kristeva, *Powers of Horror: An Essay on Abjection* (New York, 1982), pp. 1–8.

5 Ibid., p. 65, italics in the original.

6 Ibid.

7 Émile Durkheim, *The Division of Labour in Society*, with an introduction by Lewis Coser, trans. W. D. Halls (London, 1994), pp. 150, 162. Cf. Jean-Jacques Rousseau, 'On the Social Contract', in Jean-Jacques Rousseau, *Basic Political Writings*, trans. Donald A. Cress (Indianapolis, IN, 1988), pp. 141–227. In Book II, Ch. X, pp. 168–70, Rousseau argues, like Durkheim, that a social contract is only possible in a community that is already united by other ties.

8 Durkheim, *The Elementary Forms of the Religious Life*, pp. 17, 440. Cf. Kant, *Critique of Pure Reason*, A78–A79, B104–B105. Kant described time and space as pure forms of our mode of perceiving (A42, B59). The categories were 'pure concepts of understanding'. Empirical judgements imply that experience (which conforms to space and time) is synthesized (organized) by the understanding in conformity with the categories.

9 Durkheim, *The Elementary Forms of the Religious Life*, p. 17.

10 Ibid.

11 Ibid., pp. 127–33.

12 William Robertson Smith, *Lectures on the Religion of the Semites: First Series: The Fundamental Institutions* (London, 1974). See also Tiina Arppe, *Pyhä ja kirottu. Pahan ongelma ranskalaisessa yhteiskuntateoriassa* (Helsinki, 2000), p. 35.

13 Giorgio Agamben, *Homo sacer* (Paris, 1995), pp. 85–90. See also Arppe, *Pyhä ja kirottu*, p. 36.

14 Schmitt argued that a society is always constituted by its relations to the enemy. We must necessarily draw boundaries between us and persons, groups or societies designated as 'existentially different and alien', representing 'the other, the alien'. Today, Schmitt is also known as the inspiration for various neoconservative think tanks. Carl Schmitt, *Der Begriff des Politischen. Text 1932 mit Vorwort und drei Corollarien* (Berlin, 1991), p. 27.

15 See Y. Nandan, *The Durkheimian School: A Systematic and Comprehensive Bibliography* (Westport, CT, 1977).

16 Sigmund Freud, *Das Unbehagen an der Kultur* (Vienna, 1930); Sigmund Freud, 'Der Mann Moses und die monotheistische Religion', in Sigmund Freud, *Gesammelte Werke*, Band XVI: *Werke aus den Jahren 1932–1939* (London, 1950), pp. 101–246.

17 Sigmund Freud, *Totem and Taboo*, authorized trans. by A. A. Brill (New York, 1946), p. 26.

18 Ibid., pp. 38, 39–40.

19 Ibid., p. 49.

20 Ibid., p. 112.

21 Ibid., p. 108.

22 Ibid., p. 128.

23 Ibid., p. 127.

24 Ibid., p. 128; cf. Sigmund Freud, *Totem und Tabu*, in Sigmund Freud, *Gesammelte Werke*, Band IX (London, 1948), p. 121.

25 Sigmund Freud, *Das Unbehagen an der Kultur* (Vienna, 1930).

26 Ibid., p. 59. Cf. Freud, *Totem and Taboo*, p. 128.

27 Freud, *Das Unbehagen an der Kultur*, p. 59, my translation.

28 Ibid., p. 63, my translation.

29 Immanuel Kant, 'Mutmasslicher Anfang der Menschengeschichte', in Immanuel Kant, *Werke*, Band IV: *Schriften von 1783–1788*, ed. Ernst Cassirer (Berlin, 1922), pp. 325–42.

30 For instance, Michel Foucault assisted in the publication of Bataille's *Oeuvres complètes* and received his ideas on transgression and limit-experiences from him.

31 Georges Bataille, 'La valeur d'usage de D.A.F. de Sade', in *Oeuvres complètes* (Paris, 1970–88), vol. II, pp. 54–73.

32 Ibid., p. 58.

33 Georges Bataille, 'La structure psychologique du fascisme', in Georges Bataille, *Oeuvres complètes* (Paris, 1970–88), vol. I, pp. 339–71, at p. 346. '. . . les parties du corps, les personnes, les mots ou les actes ayant une valeur erotique suggestive; les divers processus inconscients tels que les rêves et les névroses; les nombreux éléments ou formes sociaux que la partie homogène est impuissante à assimiler: les foules, les classes guerrières, aristocratiques et misérables, les différentes sortes d'individus violents ou tout au moins refusant la règle (fous, meneurs, poètes, etc.).' According to Bataille, the Fascist state could arise when the homogeneous parts of society wanted to realize their dreams of purity and control. Heterogeneous, marginal social groups would be excluded from society under the command of a leader who was himself 'holy', that is, heterogeneous.

34 See Bataille, 'La valeur d'usage de D.A.F. de Sade', pp. 62–4.

35 Ibid., p. 59.

36 Georges Bataille, 'Non-savoir, rire et larmes', in Georges Bataille, *Oeuvres complètes* (Paris, 1970–88), vol. VIII, pp. 214–33.

37 Cf. 2 Corinthians 3:6, King James Version (KJV), www.biblestudytools. com, accessed 8 June 2016.

38 In finding these formulations, I was helped by the contribution of Mats Rosengren at the Nordic philosophical Symposium in Södertörn, 7 June 2002.

39 Georges Bataille, 'La Part maudite', in Georges Bataille, *Oeuvres complètes* (Paris, 1970–88), vol. VII, pp. 17–135, at pp. 70–79.

40 Bataille, 'La valeur d'usage de D.A.F. de Sade', pp. 62–3, my translation, italics in the original.

41 Imogen Tyler, 'Against Abjection', *Feminist Theory*, X (2009), pp. 77–98, at pp. 78–9.

42 Kristeva, *Powers of Horror*, pp. 56–63.

43 See, for instance, ibid, pp. 12–13, 74, 117.

44 A somewhat similar point is made by Christian Enzensberger in *Grösserer Versuch über den Schmutz* (Munich, 1970), p. 31, where the author, also drawing on Douglas, distinguishes between five main types of soiling:

'the dirt of excretion, of touch, of mixing, of decay and of superabundance' (*Schmutz der Aussonderung, Berührung, Vermischung, des Zerfalls und der Massenhaftigkeit*). These types of soiling issue threats against individual integrity, the understanding of the Ego as closed, untouchable, unified and demarcated.

45 Kristeva, *Powers of Horror*, p. 3.
46 Ibid., p. 107.
47 See ibid., p. 102, *à propos* Leviticus 13–14: 'The obsession of the leprous and decaying body would then be the fantasy of a self-rebirth on the part of a subject who has not introjected his mother but has incorporated a devouring mother. Phantasmatically, he is the solidary obverse of a cult of the Great Mother: a negative and demanding identification with her imaginary power. Aside from sanitary effectiveness, that is the fantasy that Levitical abominations aim at cutting back or resorbing.'
48 Thus, for instance, when Deuteronomy 22:6–7 states the prohibition to hunters, when robbing birds' nests, from taking the mother along with the young or eggs, Kristeva seizes on this as an obvious symbol of fear of incest and not as a thoroughly sensible precaution against decimating the stock (see Kristeva, *Powers of Horror*, p. 105).
49 Tyler, 'Against Abjection', p. 79.
50 Ibid., p. 81.
51 Julia Kristeva, *Strangers to Ourselves* (New York, 1991); Julia Kristeva, *Nations without Nationalism* (New York, 1993). Cf. Imogen Tyler, *Revolting Subjects: Social Abjection and Resistance in Neoliberal Britain* (London, 2013), pp. 29–35.
52 Kristeva, *Nations without Nationalism*, pp. 32–3.
53 Tyler, *Revolting Subjects*, p. 31; ibid., pp. 36–47.
54 On this, see, for instance, Kant, 'Mutmasslicher Anfang der Menschengeschichte'.
55 Durkheim, *The Elementary Forms of the Religious Life*, p. 17.
56 Steven Lukes, *Émile Durkheim: His Life and Works* (Harmondsworth, 1973), p. 447. See also pp. 7, 435–47.

7 The Civilizing Process

1 The variations can be quite unexpected. For instance, Finland was peripheral and economically underdeveloped in relation to central Europe but, perhaps due to the ready availability of fuel and clean water, daily bathing was a general phenomenon there (and earlier also in other parts

of Scandinavia). Moreover, this was *especially* the case among populations less touched by European modernity. Thus the frequency of bathing tended to increase as one moved from the southwest of the country towards the northeast. See P. Hakamies, 'Karelische Sauna', *Rehabilitácia*, xvi (1982), Supplement 26–7, pp. 17–20, at p. 18; Esko Aaltonen, 'On the Sociology of the *Sauna* of the Finnish Countryside', *Transactions of the Westermarck Society*, ii (1953), pp. 158–70, at p. 161: 'people could take a bath every weekday, as they did in Russia about the year 1000. In Finland, also, the daily bath has evidently been an ancient custom, although mentioned in the literature for the first time in the eighteenth century. A parish history from Satakunta (southwest Finland) from the year 1775 reveals that a daily bath was considered a bad habit for the aged and for children.'

2 Norbert Elias, *The Civilizing Process*, vol. i: *The History of Manners*, trans. Edmund Jephcott (Oxford, 1978); Norbert Elias, *The Civilizing Process*, vol. ii: *State Formation and Civilization*, trans. Edmund Jephcott with some notes and revisions by the author (Oxford, 1982).

3 Elias, *The Civilizing Process*, vol. i, pp. 189–91; vol. ii, p. 241.

4 Lorenz Lyttkens, *Den disciplinerade människan* (Stockholm, 1989), pp. 55–85.

5 Elias, *The Civilizing Process*, vol. i, pp. 69–70.

6 Lyttkens, *Den disciplinerade människan*, p. 59, my translation.

7 Ibid., p. 60, my translation.

8 Ibid., p. 63, my translation.

9 Ibid., pp. 48–51, my translation.

10 Elias, *The Civilizing Process*, vol. i, pp. 200–201.

11 Gerd Schwerhoff, 'Zivilisationsprozess und Geschichtswissenschaft: Norbert Elias' Forschungsparadigma in historischer Sicht', *Historische Zeitschrift*, cclxvi (1998), pp. 561–605, at pp. 570–71.

12 Ibid., p. 563.

13 *Keskiajan Turku – Det medeltida Åbo – Medieval Turku*, Tourist brochure (Turku, 2001), my translation. There is no documentation of how noisy and impulsive the medieval citizens of Åbo/Turku might have been. The cultural historian Hannu Laaksonen has, however, pointed out to the local newspaper that somewhat later, during the inauguration of the university in 1640, the inhabitants reportedly looked at the solemn procession *in silence*. Katja Kuokkanen, 'Meuhkasiko markkinaväki keskiajalla?', *Turkulainen*, 24 July 2002.

14 Elias, *The Civilizing Process*, vol. ii, p. 236. See also vol. i, p. 201: 'Wherever one opens the documents of this time, one finds the same: a life where

the structure of affects was different from our own, an existence without security, with only minimal thought for the future. Whoever did not love or hate to the utmost in this society, whoever could not stand his ground in the play of passions, could go into a monastery.'

15 Elias, *The Civilizing Process*, vol. II, pp. 236–7.

16 Ibid., p. 238.

17 Peter Englund, *Förflutenhetens landskap* (Stockholm, 1991). Published in German as Peter Englund, *Die Marx-Brothers in Petrograd. Reisen in die Landschaft der Vergangenheit* (Berlin, 1993).

18 Englund, *Förflutenhetens landskap*, p. 210. Englund makes a general reference to Gunnar Tilander, *Stång i vägg och hemlighus. Kulturhistoriska glimtar från mänsklighetens bakgårdar* (Stockholm, 1968). In that book, Tilander reproduces both the stories of Louis (p. 95) and Anne (p. 45) without mention of his sources. Hans Peter Duerr tells us that the king's son, the Duc de Bourgogne, would sometimes converse with members of the family while sitting on his night-stool – which was, however, noted down as curious, and those present would modestly turn their backs. Duerr refers to a letter by Princess Palatine Elisabeth Charlotte (Liselotte) of 5 May 1716. Hans Peter Duerr, *Nacktheit und Scham. Der Mythos vom Zivilisationsprozess*, Band I (Frankfurt a.M., 1988), p. 221.

19 Elias, *The Civilizing Process*, vol. I, p. 201.

20 Ibid., vol. II, p. 241.

21 Ibid., p. 242.

22 Ibid.

23 Dominique Laporte, *History of Shit*, trans. Nadia Benabid and Rodolphe el-Khoury, with an introduction by Rodolphe el-Khoury (Cambridge, MA, 2000).

24 Ibid., p. ix.

25 Ibid., p. 37.

26 Ibid.

27 Ibid., p. 48.

28 Ibid., p. 33; see also pp. 76–88.

29 Ibid., p. 78.

30 Katherine Ashenburg, *The Dirt on Clean: An Unsanitized History* (New York, 2007); Englund, *Förflutenhetens landskap*, pp. 207, 209–11.

31 On the use of water, see Ashenburg, *Dirt on Clean*, pp. 97–159. On urban population growth and its inconveniences, see Emily Cockayne, *Hubbub: Filth, Noise and Stench in England, 1600–1770* (New Haven, CT, and London, 2007).

32 See Ludvig Nordström, 'Ur "Lort-Sverige"', *Res Publica*, LVII (2002), pp. 37–41.

33 We are told that in the traditional peasant household, the tables, chairs and benches were washed every Saturday and the dining table was wiped clean after each meal, while the floors were swept at least once a day. When major cleaning was undertaken, which was at least twice or thrice a year (but more frequently in the bedrooms), windows were cleaned, dust and cobwebs were removed from ceilings and floors were scrubbed clean with soap and water. Kustaa Vilkuna, *Varsinais-Suomen kansanrakennukset. Varsinais-Suomen historia*, vol. II/1 (Porvoo, 1938), p. 21; Vilkuna's description follows the account of J. F. Huukanen from the parish of Taivassalo in 1889.

34 Johann Konrad Eberlein, 'Abschweifungen: Der Mensch, sein Abfall und die Kunst', in *Abfallmoderne. Zu den Schmutzrändern der Kultur*, ed. Anselm Wagner (Vienna, 2011), pp. 9–15, at p. 11.

35 Duerr, *Nacktheit und Scham*, p. 241.

36 Henry Nygård, *Bara ett ringa obehag? Avfall och renhållning i de finländska städernas profylaktiska strategier 1830–1930* (Åbo, 2004), pp. 110–11.

37 Ibid., p. 301.

38 Elias, *The Civilizing Process*, vol. I, p. 72.

39 Schwerhoff, 'Zivilisationsprozess und Geschichtswissenschaft', p. 576.

40 Duerr, *Nacktheit und Scham*, pp. 216, 241.

41 Elias, *The Civilizing Process*, vol. I, pp. 199–201, cf. Schwerhoff, 'Zivilisationsprozess und Geschichtswissenschaft', p. 577.

42 Duerr, *Nacktheit und Scham*, pp. 227–41; on nakedness outside European cultures, see pp. 135–49.

43 Ibid., p. 335.

44 Duerr's illustrations also show a great deal of variety across cultures, situations, sexes and age groups, and his choice of material from outside Europe looks unsystematic. Cf. Schwerhoff, 'Zivilisationsprozess und Geschichtswissenschaft', p. 565.

45 Duerr, *Nacktheit und Scham*, p. 211.

46 Ibid., pp. 211–12.

47 Ibid., p. 22; see also Tilander, *Stång i vägg och hemlighus*, pp. 96–8.

48 'If ye case require that thou muste name some shamefull member, thou muste signifye it by some modestius disguysing. Furthermore if any thing chañce that may trouble the heart, as yf anye men do speake of vomiting, of a iakes [= jakes], or of a turde, he must pray him that it displease not his eares.' In Desiderius Erasmus, *The Ciuilitie of Childehode*, trans. Thomas

Paynell (London, 1560), n.p. Cf.: 'Si res exigat, vt aliquod membrum pudendum nominetur, circumitione verecûda rem notet. Rursus si quid inciderit, quod auditori nauseam ciere possit, velut si quis narret vomitum, aut latrinam, aut oletum, praefetur honorem auribus.' In Desiderius Erasmus, *De civilitate morum puerilium* (Lugduni, 1536), fol. 12v.

49 Duerr, *Nacktheit und Scham*, p. 224.

50 Ibid., pp. 221–2.

51 Duerr relates (ibid., p. 221) how the Duc de Vendôme, a cousin of Louis XIV, received an envoy of the Duke of Parma sitting on his night-stool. His guest's great surprise was further increased when Vendôme got up and wiped his behind in full sight of the envoy, who was the bishop of Parma. The bishop broke off the negotiations immediately, left and vowed never to return. Duerr refers to Alfred Franklin, *La civilité*, vol. II (Paris, 1908), p. 34. The popular account by Tilander, *Stång i vägg och hemlighus*, pp. 95–6, re-tells this event, but the author is (characteristically) quite silent about the guest's reactions, thereby conveying the misleading impression that nothing was amiss with the Duke's behaviour.

52 Ulrik Langen, *Den afmægtige – en biografi om Christian 7* (Copenhagen, 2008), p. 272, my translation.

8 Ambiguities of Self-discipline and the Campaign for Civilization

1 Hans Peter Duerr, *Nacktheit und Scham. Der Mythos vom Zivilisationsprozess*, Band I (Frankfurt a.M., 1988), pp. 227–33.

2 Ibid., pp. 224–5.

3 Ibid., Ch. 8 (pp. 135–49).

4 Ibid., p. 135, my translation.

5 Ibid., p. 133.

6 Helena Hänninen, *Puhtauden yhteiskunnallis-sosiaalisia ulottuvuuksia. Henkilökohtainen siisteys ja puhtaudenpito Keski-Suomessa noin 1890–1930*. MA dissertation, University of Jyväskylä (1985), p. 73. On exoticism concerning Russian naked bathing in the eighteenth century, see Duerr, *Nacktheit und Scham*, pp. 129–31.

7 Hänninen, *Puhtauden yhteiskunnallis-sosiaalisia ulottuvuuksia*, p. 72.

8 On mixed bathing, see Esko Aaltonen, 'On the Sociology of the *Sauna* of the Finnish Countryside', *Transactions of the Westermarck Society*, II (1953), pp. 158–70; P. Leimu, 'Sauna as a Socializing Instrument',

Rehabilitácia, XVI, Supplement 26–7 (1982), pp. 12–14, at p. 12. Leimu also notes: 'It was, however, quite clear that different sexes did not bathe together in whatever combination: for instance young marri[age]able women and men never bathed together.'

9 Joseph [Giuseppe] Acerbi, *Travels through Sweden, Finland, and Lapland, to the North Cape in the Years 1798 and 1799*, vol. I (London, 1802), p. 297.

10 Gerd Schwerhoff, 'Zivilisationsprozess und Geschichtswissenschaft: Norbert Elias' Forschungsparadigma in historischer Sicht', *Historische Zeitschrift*, CCLXVI (1998), pp. 599–600, points out that Elias presents his own work explicitly as an empirically verified historical thesis and not as an ideal construct or framework for further research.

11 Christer Winberg, 'Några anteckningar om historisk antropologi', *Historisk tidskrift*, CVIII (1988), pp. 1–29, at p. 19, my translation. The last quote (with italics in the original) is cited from a review, by Sven B. Ek, of J. Frykman and O. Löfgren, ed., *Den kultiverade människan* (Lund, 1979).

12 I was first made aware of the importance of this fact by Dr Solveig Sjöberg-Pietarinen, in discussion, 20 March 2002.

13 Cf. also *recht* (German), *droit* (French), *pravyj* (Russian), *oikea* (Finnish) and *parem* (Estonian). Cf. further some Swedish colloquialisms: *grannhanden* 'the pretty (= right) hand' (S. Sjöberg-Pietarinen, oral communication, 20 March 2002); *taga skeden i vacker hand* 'grab the spoon with one's beautiful (= right) hand'.

14 Martti Grönfors, 'Institutional Non-marriage in the Finnish Roma Community and Its Relationship to Rom Traditional Law', in *Gypsy Law: Romani Legal Traditions and Culture*, ed. Walter O. Weyrauch (Berkeley, CA, 2001), pp. 149–69, at pp. 149–50, fn. 2: 'For the Finnish Roma, if something is ritually unclean it is also then practically unclean. If something is ritually unclean, it cannot be cleansed at all by any means, whereas if something is ritually pure but practically unclean it can be cleaned, for example, by washing in the normal manner. If, for example, a coffee cup (inherently clean, i.e. ritually pure) enters a ritually unclean surface it cannot be cleaned by any means.'

15 Ibid., p. 158, fn. 19: 'The tabooed garments (e.g. bras, men's shirts, and underclothes) could not be referred to in speech . . . the clothes of each generation and gender were washed separately. In addition "clean" things (like table cloths and face towels) could not be washed with "dirty" things (like clothes).'

16 Ibid., p. 157, fn. 18.

17 Ibid.

18 Gunilla Lundgren and Aljosha Taikon, *Aljosha – zigenarhövdingens pojke* (Stockholm, 1998), pp. 68–9.

19 Peter Englund, *Förflutenhetens landskap* (Stockholm, 1991), p. 208.

20 Ibid., p. 207.

21 Jonas Frykman, 'Hel och ren. Kropp och tanke hos bönder och borgare', in *Den kultiverade människan*, ed. J. Frykman and O. Löfgren (Lund, 1979), pp. 131–220.

22 Clara Puranen, 'En anslående fest', in *Sagalund – 'min kostsamma leksak'*, ed. Li Näse, Sagalunds Museum (Kimito, 2000), pp. 8–43, at p. 20, my translation.

23 Hänninen, *Puhtauden yhteiskunnallis-sosiaalisia ulottuvuuksia*, p. 94.

24 Already around the year 1200, in the history of Denmark known as *Gesta danorum*, chronicler Saxo Grammaticus mentions the habit of picking one's teeth and eating the food fragments as a mark of lowly birth. This is included in the story of Amleth (the source of Shakespeare's *Hamlet*), which is based on earlier folklore. Saxo Grammaticus, *Danica historia libris XVI*, ed. Philippus Lonicerus (Francofurti ad Moenum, 1576), Book III, p. 48.

25 Desiderius Erasmus, *The Ciuilitie of Childehode*, trans. Thomas Paynell (London, 1560), n.p.

26 Jerzy Faryno, 'Neskol'ko obščih soobraženij po povodu konceptov "grjaznyj/čistyj"', *Studia Litteraria Polono-Slavica*, IV (1999), pp. 59–62. By kissing, the misbegotten loaf of bread is literally welcomed back into the sphere of the edible. The kiss may be seen as a friendly greeting but also as confirmation of the fact that nothing has happened to encroach on the bread's purity.

27 Erasmus, *The Ciuilitie of Childehode*, n.p.

28 Norbert Elias, *The Civilizing Process*, vol. I: *The History of Manners*, trans. Edmund Jephcott (Oxford, 1978), pp. 69–70.

29 Irja Sahlberg, 'Byggnadsskick och heminredning', in *Kimitobygdens historia*, vol. II (Ekenäs, 1982), pp. 61–139, at p. 107, my translation.

30 Kirsti Suolinna, oral communication, 17 November 2004.

31 On early campaigns for personal cleanliness in the U.S. see Katherine Ashenburg, *The Dirt on Clean: An Unsanitized History* (New York, 2007), pp. 200–227.

32 Nordström, quoted in Per Svensson, *Svenska hem. En bok om hur vi bor och varför* (Stockholm, 2002), p. 164, my translation.

33 Ashenburg, *The Dirt on Clean*, p. 201.

34 See also Roger Fayet, 'Moderne Reinigung, postmoderne Kompostierung. Über ein abfalltheoretisches Modell und die

eigentlichen Signaturen zweier Zeitalter', in *Verlangen nach Reinheit oder Lust auf Schmutz? Gestaltungskonzepte zwischen rein und unrein*, ed. Roger Fayet (Vienna, 2003), pp. 15–40, at p. 15, and his suggestion that 'the real signature of the Modern is the purifying tendency, the real signature of the Postmodern is, on the other hand, the tendency to "compost"' (my translation); and Stanislaus von Moos, 'Das Prinzip Toilette. Über Loos, Le Corbusier und die Reinlichkeit', in *Verlangen nach Reinheit oder Lust auf Schmutz? Gestaltungskonzepte zwischen rein und unrein*, ed. Roger Fayet (Vienna, 2003), pp. 41–58, at p. 42, describing 'bath, cleanliness, purification' as 'obsessions of the Modern' (my translation); and further Elsa Törne [Elna Tenow], *Renhet. En häfstång för den enskilde och samhället* (Stockholm, 1906), pp. 3–4: 'I have been trying to show that dirt exerts a crippling power over our societies, and that we are all more or less slaves under it: slaves or martyrs. Above all I have found that successively lifting up one social group after another insofar as they themselves manage to make their demands effective is a far too slow way of reaching the goal. Instead I have wanted to point to *one single line* capable of running through all levels of society like nothing else – namely *the line of cleanliness*' . . . 'the same shining cleanliness to all, now only on offer to the relatively low number of the so-called well-to-do members of society.' (My translation, italics in the original.)

35 Ashenburg, *The Dirt on Clean*, p. 248. The first quote is from William M. Handy, *The Science of Culture* (1923), 1:58.

36 *Kvinnans bokskatt*, ed. Ingrid Norden (Stockholm, 1913), quoted from Svensson, *Svenska hem*, p. 109, my translation.

37 Susan Strasser, *Waste and Want: A Social History of Trash* (New York, 1999), p. 174.

38 G.V.L., 1908. Ihminen on eläin. *Terveydenhoitolehti*, xx/11 (1908), p. 179, quoted from Helena Hänninen, *Puhtauden yhteiskunnallis-sosiaalisia ulottuvuuksia. Henkilökohtainen siisteys ja puhtaudenpito Keski-Suomessa noin 1890–1930*, MA dissertation, University of Jyväskylä (1985), p. 39.

39 Arvid Järnefelt, *Mitt uppvaknande* (Helsingfors, 1894), pp. 30–32.

40 Hänninen, *Puhtauden yhteiskunnallis-sosiaalisia ulottuvuuksia*, p. 37. Hänninen has searched through several annual volumes of the Finnish magazine *Terveydenhoitolehti*.

41 Metsätähti, 1908, 'Siveelisyydestä'. *Terveydenhoitolehti*, xx/11 (1908), quoted from Hänninen, *Puhtauden yhteiskunnallis-sosiaalisia ulottuvuuksia*, p. 36, my translation.

42 Annie Furuhjelm, *Den stigande oron* (Helsingfors, 1935), pp. 186–7, my translation.

43 Ibid., p. 187, my translation.

44 Strasser, *Waste and Want*, p. 137, quoting H. de B. Parsons, *The Disposal of Municipal Refuse* (New York, 1906), p. 6.

45 Ibid., p. 139, quoting David Ward, *Poverty, Ethnicity, and the American City, 1840–1925: Changing Conceptions of the Slum and the Ghetto* (Cambridge, 1989), pp. 17–18, 33–4, 77.

46 Strasser, *Waste and Want*, p. 139.

47 Schwerhoff, 'Zivilisationsprozess und Geschichtswissenschaft', pp. 601, 584.

48 Ibid., p. 595.

49 Lorenz Lyttkens, *Den disciplinerade människan* (Stockholm, 1989), p. 63.

PART III: SETTLING ACCOUNTS WITH MATTER

1 Jean-Paul Sartre, *Sketch for a Theory of Emotions*, trans. Philip Mairet (London and New York, 1962), p. 39.

2 Luke 12:25–6 (NRSV).

9 Between Facts and Practices

1 Simone Weil, *Lectures on Philosophy*, trans. Hugh Price, with an introduction by Peter Winch (Cambridge, 1993), p. 52.

2 Tim Ingold, *Making: Anthropology, Archaeology, Art and Architecture* (London, 2013), p. 27.

3 Arjun Appadurai, 'Introduction: Commodities and the Politics of Value', in *The Social Life of Things: Commodities in Cultural Perspective*, ed. Arjun Appadurai (Cambridge, 1988), p. 3.

4 Ibid., p. 4.

5 Marx argued that the fetishism of commodities was an illusion created by the market mechanism, whereby it could, for instance, appear that the 'value' of a commodity fluctuated without the object itself undergoing any change. Thus he could protest, 'So far no chemist has ever discovered exchange-value either in a pearl or a diamond' (Karl Marx, *Capital*, vol. I, trans. Samuel Moore and Edward Aveling (New York, 1967), p. 83). But in his discussion of the fetishism of commodities, Marx operates with a notion of 'value' closely connected with *exchange* value and therefore fully

applicable only under conditions of capitalism, that is, in a life form where the dominating mode of production is that of producing for a market (on the fetishism of commodities, ibid., pp. 71–83).

6 Appadurai, 'Introduction', p. 5, italics in the original.

7 Marx, *Capital*, vol. i, p. 36, fn. 4, attributed to Butler.

8 Göran Torrkulla, *Om mötet med konst som en dialektik mellan tilltal, gensvar och ansvar, eller om konsten som en dialogskapande vägkost.* Lecture manuscript, Åbo Akademi University (Åbo, 2004).

9 Le Corbusier, *L'Art décoratif d'aujourd'hui, 1925* (Paris, 2008), p. 191, my translation.

10 John Searle asks basically the same question in the context of materialist philosophy of mind. His question is how the world, being essentially devoid of meaning, can include meanings. John Searle, *Minds, Brains and Science* (Cambridge, MA, 1984), at p. 13.

11 Ludwig Wittgenstein, *Philosophical Investigations*, ed. G.E.M. Anscombe and G. H. von Wright, trans. G.E.M. Anscombe (Oxford, 1953), i:§251.

12 Ingold, *Making*, p. 70.

13 Martin Heidegger, 'The Thing', in Martin Heidegger, *Poetry, Language, Thought*, trans. A. Hofstadter (New York, 1971), pp. 163–84, at p. 165; Martin Heidegger, 'Das Ding', in Martin Heidegger, *Gesamtausgabe*, Band vii: *Vorträge und Aufsätze* (Frankfurt a.M., 2000), pp. 167–187, at p. 168 [159].

14 Heidegger, 'The Thing', pp. 172, 179; Heidegger, 'Das Ding', pp. 176 [167], 182 [174]; Ingold, *Making*, pp. 85–6.

15 Martin Heidegger, *Being and Time*, trans. John Macquarrie and Edward Robinson (Oxford, 2001), p. 101 [71].

16 Karl Marx, 'Thesen über Feuerbach', in Karl Marx and Friedrich Engels, *Werke* (= MEW), Band iii (Berlin, 1978), pp. 5–7, Thesis 9, p. 7, my translation.

17 Marx, 'Thesen über Feuerbach', Thesis 1, p. 5, my translation, italics in the original.

18 'Dialectical materialism' seems to be a later designation of Marxist philosophy, but it certainly captures an important strand of what Marx was doing.

19 Karl Marx and Friedrich Engels, 'Die deutsche Ideologie', in Karl Marx and Friedrich Engels, *Werke* (= MEW), Band iii (Berlin, 1978), pp. 9–521, at p. 30.

20 The available translation on the Internet renders the last phrase, 'gegenständliche Tätigkeit', as 'objective activity', which obscures the implied reference to '*Gegenstände*' (concrete things) as opposed to

'objects'. See Karl Marx, 'Theses on Feuerbach', trans. Cyril Smith, 1978, at www.marxists.org, accessed 8 June 2016.

21 Jakob Meløe, 'Steder', *Hammarn*, 3 (1995), pp. 6–13.

22 Jakob Meløe, 'The Two Landscapes of Northern Norway', *Inquiry*, XXXI (1988), pp. 387–401, at p. 393, italics in the original.

23 Meløe, 'Steder', p. 8. For translations of *Zeug*, see Martin Heidegger, *Being and Time*, p. 97 [68], fn. 1 and Martin Heidegger, *Being and Time: A Translation of 'Sein und Zeit'*, trans. Joan Stambaugh (Albany, NY, 1996), p. 64 [68].

24 Meløe, 'Steder', p. 8.

25 Ibid.; see also Heidegger, *Being and Time*, p. 97 [68]: 'Taken strictly, there "is" no such thing as *an* equipment. To the Being of any equipment there always belongs a totality of equipment, in which it can be this equipment that it is.'

26 Kaisa Pennanen, 'Humanistisesta paikan tulkinnasta ja lian käsitteestä', *Alue ja ympäristö*, III/1 (2004), pp. 55–61.

27 Meløe, 'The Two Landscapes of Northern Norway', p. 393, italics in the original.

28 Weil, *Lectures on Philosophy*, p. 52.

29 Ibid., p. 50.

30 Marx, 'Theses on Feuerbach', Theses 2 and 9, pp. 5, 7, translation modified by me.

31 Philosopher Peter Winch has this in mind when he states, 'Reality is not what gives language sense. What is real and what is unreal shows itself *in* the sense that language has'. In other words, we learn the meaning of the concept of *reality* by learning the kinds of distinction actually made when this concept is used in language. Winch, 'Understanding a Primitive Society', in Peter Winch, *Ethics and Action* (London, 1972), pp. 8–49, at p. 12.

32 Jonas Ahlskog and Olli Lagerspetz, 'Language-games and Relativism: On Cora Diamond's Reading of Peter Winch', *Philosophical Investigations*, XXXVIII (2015), pp. 293–315, at p. 295. See also Peter Winch, *Trying to Make Sense* (Oxford, 1987), p. 42.

33 Paraphrasing Peter Winch, private communication, Spring 1991.

10 To Dress and to Keep

1 Martin Heidegger, *Being and Time*, trans. John Macquarrie and Edward Robinson (Oxford, 2001), p. 235 [191].

2 Edwyn Bevan, *Hellenism and Christianity* (London, 1921), p. 154, quoted in Katherine Ashenburg, *The Dirt on Clean: An Unsanitized History* (New York, 2007), p. 279.

3 Yury Tynyanov, *Young Pushkin: A Novel*, trans. Anna Kurkina Rush (New York, 2008), quoted in Timo Suni, 'Tšuhnalainen automenodi', in *Toisten Suomi*, ed. Hannes Sihvo (Jyväskylä, 2001), pp. 196–242, at p. 210, my translation.

4 Jerzy Faryno, 'Neskol'ko obščih soobraženij po povodu konceptov "grjaznyj/čistyj"', *Studia Litteraria Polono-Slavica*, IV (1999), pp. 59–62.

5 Genesis 1:31 (NRSV).

6 Heidegger, *Being and Time*, p. 135 [102].

7 Vilppu Vuorela, *Kitchen Dreams*, exh. cat., Galleria Spectro, Turku (Turku, 2003).

8 Leena Pitkänen, 'Sottakeittiö pelasti', *Turkulainen*, 23 August 2003, p. 12, my translation.

9 Vuorela, *Kitchen Dreams*; Susanne Sperring, 'Han dokumenterade sitt smutsiga kök', *Åbo Underrättelser*, 14 August 2003.

10 Susan Strasser, in *Waste and Want: A Social History of Trash* (New York, 1999), uses 'The Stewardship of Objects' as the title of her first chapter (pp. 21–67). A similar idea was noted, with quite an opposite emphasis, by Le Corbusier who accused the traditionalists of his own time of turning 'our home into a museum or temple full of votive gifts and our soul into a kind of museum keeper, a custodian'. Le Corbusier [Charles-Edouard Jeanneret], *L'Art décoratif d'aujourd'hui, 1925* (Paris, 2008), p. 191, my translation (also quoted in Stanislaus von Moos, 'Das Prinzip Toilette. Über Loos, Le Corbusier und die Reinlichkeit', in *Verlangen nach Reinheit oder Lust auf Schmutz? Gestaltungskonzepte zwischen rein und unrein*, ed. Roger Fayet (Vienna, 2003), pp. 41–58, at p. 55).

11 Strasser, *Waste and Want*, p. 22.

12 Ningtsu Malmqvist, *Ningtsus kinesiska kokbok* (Stockholm, 1988), pp. 12–13.

13 John Scanlan, *On Garbage* (London, 2005) pp. 22–3; *The Concise Oxford Dictionary of Current English*, pp. 1447–8 (waste).

14 Genesis 2:15 (KJV). Alternative translation (NRSV): 'The Lord God took the man and put him in the garden of Eden to till it and keep it.'

15 Strasser, *Waste and Want*, p. 187.

16 Oswald Spengler, *Der Mensch und die Technik* (Munich, 1931), pp. 28–30, argues that the tool and the human hand appeared at the same time in

history, and further, that the differentiation between *using* a tool and *making* or modifying it gave rise to the possibility of choosing between tools, a kind of freedom that Spengler identifies as specifically human.

17 Henry Nygård, *Bara ett ringa obehag? Avfall och renhållning i de finländska städernas profylaktiska strategier 1830–1930* (Åbo, 2004).

18 Ibid., p. 109, my translation.

19 Strasser, *Waste and Want*, p. 29.

20 *The Concise Oxford Dictionary of Current English*, pp. 307 (debris), 494 (garbage), 646 (junk), 697 (litter), 1074 (rubbish), 1327 (thrash), 1359 (trash).

21 Cyrille Harpet, *Du déchet: Philosophie des immondices. Corps, ville, industrie* (Paris – Montréal, 1998), pp. 50–51.

22 Johann Georg Krünitz, Ökonomisch-technologische *Enzyklopädie*, Band I (1773), elektronische Ausgabe der Universitätsbibliothek Trier, www.kruenitz.uni-trier.de/1773, accessed 8 June 2016, p. 43.

23 *Svenska Akademins ordbok (SAOB)*, http://g3.spraakdata.gu.se/osa/index. html, accessed 8 June 2016, A165: 'affall'.

24 'Article L541-1-1 Créé par Ordonnance n°2010-1579 du 17 décembre 2010' art. 2: 'Au sens du présent chapitre, on entend par: Déchet: toute substance ou tout objet, ou plus généralement tout bien meuble, dont le détenteur se défait ou dont il a l'intention ou l'obligation de se défaire'. www.legifrance. gouv.fr, accessed 5 May 2016.

25 According to 'Directive 2006/12/EC of the European Parliament and of the Council of 5 April 2006 on waste', '"waste" shall mean any substance or object in the categories set out in Annex I which the holder discards or intends or is required to discard' (Article 1). *Official Journal of the European Union*, 27.4.2006, L114/9, at http://eur-lex.europa.eu/legal-content, accessed 6 May 2016.

26 'Loi ° 75–633 du 15 juillet 1975 relative à l'élimination des déchets et à la récupération des matériaux', *Journal officiel de la République française* (16 July 1975), p. 7279. Available at www.legifrance.gouv.fr, accessed 5 July 2017.

27 Cf. 'Directive 2006/12/EC of the European Parliament and of the Council of 5 April 2006 on waste', Article 8: 'Member States shall take the necessary measures to ensure that any holder of waste: (a) has it handled by a private or public waste collector or by an undertaking which carries out the operations listed in Annex II A or II B; or (b) recovers or disposes of it himself in accordance with the provisions of this Directive.'

28 'Article L541-1-1 Créé par Ordonnance n°2010-1579 du 17 décembre 2010', art. 4; citing Waste Framework Directive 2008/98/EC.

29 See also the 'waste theoretic model' by Fayet, with the starting point that waste is something from which we wish to distance ourselves. Roger Fayet, 'Moderne Reinigung, postmoderne Kompostierung. Über ein abfalltheoretisches Modell und die eigentlichen Signaturen zweier Zeitalter', in *Verlangen nach Reinheit oder Lust auf Schmutz? Gestaltungskonzepte zwischen rein und unrein*, ed. Roger Fayet (Vienna, 2003), pp. 15–40, at pp. 18–21.

30 Pia Maria Ahlbäck, *Energy, Heterotopia, Dystopia: George Orwell, Michel Foucault and the Twentieth Century Environmental Imagination* (Åbo, 2001), especially pp. 170–77.

31 Ibid., p. 173.

32 Annie Furuhjelm, *Den stigande oron* (Helsingfors, 1935), p. 186.

33 *Lördag*, Swedish for Saturday, is etymologically connected with *löddra*, 'to make foam (e.g. with soap)'. Saturday was the day for cleaning and washing.

34 Ludwig Wittgenstein, *Culture and Value*, ed. G. H. von Wright and Heikki Nyman, trans. Peter Winch (Chicago, IL, 1984), p. 71e.

11 What Is Mine and What Is Someone Else's

1 Mark 10:8 (NRSV).

2 This is not to say that there may not be cases of 'symmetrical' uses of 'here', 'over there', and so on. One case would be when I point to my current position on a map. 'I am there' is here used similarly to 'Camilla is there'. The word 'I' sometimes has the character of an indexical and sometimes of a referring expression. See G.E.M. Anscombe, 'The First Person', in G.E.M Anscombe, *Collected Philosophical Papers*, vol. II (Minneapolis, MN, 1981), pp. 21–36.

3 As Peter Winch points out, to treat a person 'as an object' is not the same thing as treating *an object* 'as an object'. A person who stands in the way and is physically pushed aside is treated as an object but she is also, in a sense, defiled, which cannot be said of a stone removed from a piece of waste ground. Peter Winch, *Simone Weil: 'The Just Balance'* (Cambridge, 1989), p. 154.

4 For a model of the relation between social class relations and soiling, see Christian Enzensberger, *Grösserer Versuch über den Schmutz* (Munich, 1970), pp. 50–53, 70–77. On Simone Weil's idea of 'the power to refuse', see Winch, *Simone Weil*, pp. 102–19.

5 Jami Jokinen, 'Liasta näkyy vain osa', *Turkulainen*, 4 June 2003.

6 Anscombe, 'The First Person'.

7 Fyodor Dostoevsky, *The Brothers Karamazov* (New York, 1976), Book
9, Ch. VI. Ludwig Wittgenstein apparently has this scene in mind
in his 'Remarks on Frazer's *Golden Bough*', in Ludwig Wittgenstein,
Philosophical Occasions 1912–1951, ed. James Klagge and Alfred
Nordmann (Indianapolis, IN, 1993), pp. 115–55, at p. 155.

8 Norbert Elias, *The Civilizing Process*, vol. II: *State Formation and
Civilization*, trans. Edmund Jephcott, with some notes and revisions
by the author (Oxford, 1982).

9 I am here disregarding the fact that mucus, food and so on in the other's
mouth would be disturbing, just as they would be in my own mouth.

10 Jaan Kross, *The Czar's Madman: A Novel*, trans. Anselm Hollo (New York,
1993), p. 65.

11 See Hildur Kalman and Katarina Andersson, 'Framing of Intimate Care
in Home Care Services', *European Journal of Social Work*, XVII/3 (2014),
pp. 402–14.

12 Information from Prof. Hildur Kalman, email, 1 June 2016.

13 According to an estimate of professionals, 80 per cent of the work at
nursing homes goes to feeding, washing and administering the various
body discharges of patients; Gertrud Rückert, 'Gedanken einer alten
Frau zur allerletzten Seite der ZEIT', *Die Zeit*, 6 December 1994. Compare
with the account by Lapcic of the conditions at a hospice: 'Doctors and
nurses had time to administer each and every medicine, but no time for
talk', where the medicalization of patient–staff interaction is evidently just
another facet of the anonymous character of the situation. M. Lapcic, 'Die
Federn Richtung Himmel steigen lassen', *Frankfurter Allgemeine Zeitung*,
27 October 2014.

14 Jochen Temsch, 'Das wird schon wieder werden', *Die Zeit*, 25 November
1994.

15 Ibid.

16 Rückert, 'Gedanken einer alten Frau'.

17 Ibid.

18 Ibid.

19 Julia Kristeva, *Powers of Horror: An Essay on Abjection* (New York, 1982).

20 Ulrika Wolf-Knuts, 'Liktvättning', *Skärgård*, VII (1984), pp. 35–9, at
p. 39.

21 Ibid., p. 37.

22 Primo Levi, 'If This Is a Man', in Primo Levi, *If This Is a Man* and *The
Truce*, trans. Stuart Woolf (London, 2007), pp. 15–179, at p. 46.

23 Alexander Solzhenitsyn, *One Day in the Life of Ivan Denisovich*, trans. Ralph Parker (New York, 1963), www.kkoworld.com accessed 31 May 2016, at p. 12.

24 On asceticism, see Jerzy Faryno, 'Neskol'ko obščih soobraženij po povodu konceptov "grjaznyj/čistyj"', *Studia Litteraria Polono-Slavica*, IV (1999), pp. 59–62.; on holy fools, see Ewa Majewska Thompson, *Understanding Russia: The Holy Fool in Russian Culture* (Lanham, MD, 1987).

25 Pierre Hadot, *Plotinus or the Simplicity of Vision* (Chicago, IL, 1998).

26 Matthew 15:10–20 (NRSV).

27 Genesis 2:15; Genesis 1:28 (NRSV).

28 Genesis 17:5 (NRSV).

29 Egon Friedell, *Kulturgeschichte des Altertums. Leben und Legende der vorchristlichen Seele*, Band I (Zürich, 1936), p. 3, my translation.

30 Ludwig Wittgenstein, *Notebooks, 1914–1916*, ed. G. H. von Wright and G.E.M. Anscombe, trans. G.E.M. Anscombe (New York, 1961), p. 83e.

BIBLIOGRAPHY

Aaltonen, Esko, 'On the Sociology of the *Sauna* of the Finnish Countryside',
  Transactions of the Westermarck Society, II (1953), pp. 158–70

Acerbi, Joseph [Giuseppe], *Travels through Sweden, Finland, and Lapland,
  to the North Cape in the Years 1798 and 1799*, vol. I (London, 1802)

Agamben, Giorgio, *Homo sacer* (Paris, 1995)

Ahlbäck, Pia Maria, *Energy, Heterotopia, Dystopia: George Orwell, Michel
  Foucault and the Twentieth Century Environmental Imagination*
  (Åbo, 2001)

Ahlskog, Jonas, and Olli Lagerspetz, 'Language-games and Relativism:
  On Cora Diamond's Reading of Peter Winch', *Philosophical Investigations*,
  XXXVIII (2015), pp. 293–315

Anscombe, G.E.M., 'The First Person', in G.E.M Anscombe, *Collected
  Philosophical Papers*, vol. II (Minneapolis, MN, 1981), pp. 21–36

——, 'On Brute Facts', in G.E.M. Anscombe, *Collected Philosophical Papers*,
  vol. III (Minneapolis, 1981), pp. 22–5

Appadurai, Arjun, 'Introduction: Commodities and the Politics of Value',
  in *The Social Life of Things: Commodities in Cultural Perspective*,
  ed. Arjun Appadurai (Cambridge, 1988)

Aristotle, *Generation of Animals*, trans. A. L. Peck (Cambridge, MA, 1946)

——, *Metaphysics*, trans. W. D. Ross, in *The Works of Aristotle*, ed. W. D. Ross,
  vol. VIII (Oxford, 1960)

——, *Politics*, trans. Benjamin Jowett (Oxford, 1938)

——, *Problems*, Books I–XXI, trans. W. S. Hett (London, 1961)

Arppe, Tiina, *Pyhä ja kirottu. Pahan ongelma ranskalaisessa yhteiskuntateoriassa*
  (Helsinki, 2000)

'Article L541-1-1 Créé par Ordonnance n°2010-1579 du 17 décembre 2010',
  www.legifrance.gouv.fr, accessed 5 May 2016

Ashenburg, Katherine, *The Dirt on Clean: An Unsanitized History*
  (New York, 2007)

Baker, Lynne Rudder, 'A Metaphysics of Ordinary Things and Why We Need It', *Philosophy*, LXXXIII (2008), pp. 5–24

Bataille, Georges, 'La structure psychologique du fascisme', in Georges Bataille, *Oeuvres complètes* (Paris, 1970–88), vol. I, pp. 339–71

——, 'La valeur d'usage de D.A.F. de Sade', in Georges Bataille, *Oeuvres complètes* (Paris, 1970–88), vol. II, pp. 54–73

——, 'La Part maudite', in Georges Bataille, *Oeuvres complètes* (Paris, 1970–88), vol. VII, pp. 17–135

——, 'Non-savoir, rire et larmes', in Georges Bataille, *Oeuvres complètes* (Paris, 1970–88), vol. VIII, pp. 214–33

Bauman, Zygmunt, *Postmodernity and Its Discontents* (Cambridge, 1997)

Bible, King James Version (KJV), www.biblestudytools.com, accessed 8 June 2016

——, New Revised Standard Version (NRSV), www.biblestudytools.com, accessed 8 June 2016

Björkman, Nina, 'Gränsfallsbilder', *Hufvudstadsbladet*, 13 April 2002, p. 14

Blackstock, Colin, 'Cleaner Cleans Up Hirst's Ashtray Art', *The Guardian*, 19 October 2001, at www.theguardian.com

Cockayne, Emily, *Hubbub: Filth, Noise and Stench in England, 1600–1770* (New Haven, CT, and London, 2007)

Collingwood, R. G., 'Preliminary Discussion: The Idea of a Philosophy of Something, and, in Particular, a Philosophy of History (1927)', in R. G. Collingwood, *The Idea of History, With Lectures, 1926–1928*, revd edn, ed. Jan van der Dussen (Oxford, 2005), pp. 335–58

Comte-Sponville, André, *A Small Treatise on the Great Virtues: The Uses of Philosophy in Everyday Life* (New York, 2003)

The Concise Oxford Dictionary of Current English, ed. H. W. Fowler and F. G. Fowler (Oxford, 1956)

Cox, Rosie, 'Introduction', in *Dirt: New Geographies of Cleanliness and Contamination*, ed. Ben Campkin and Rosie Cox (London, 2007)

Dagognet, François, *Rematérialiser. Matières et matérialismes* (Paris, 1985)

'Directive 2006/12/EC of the European Parliament and of the Council of 5 April 2006 on Waste', *Official Journal of the European Union*, 27 April 2006, L114/9, at http://eur-lex.europa.eu/legal-content, accessed 6 May 2016

Dostoevsky, Fyodor, *The Brothers Karamazov* [1880] (New York, 1976)

Douglas, Mary, *Purity and Danger: An Analysis of Concepts of Pollution and Taboo* (Harmondsworth, 1970)

Duerr, Hans Peter, *Nacktheit und Scham. Der Mythos vom Zivilisationsprozess*, Band 1 (Frankfurt a.M., 1988)

Durkheim, Émile, *The Division of Labour in Society*, trans. W. D. Halls with an
     introduction by Lewis Coser, (London, 1994)
——, *The Elementary Forms of the Religious Life* (London, 1968)
Eberlein, Johann Konrad, 'Abschweifungen: Der Mensch, sein Abfall und die
     Kunst', in *Abfallmoderne. Zu den Schmutzrändern der Kultur*, ed. Anselm
     Wagner (Vienna, 2011), pp. 9–15
Eddington, A. S., *The Nature of the Physical World* (New York, 1929)
Egyptian Book of the Dead, ed. E. A. Wallis Budge (New York, 1967)
Elias, Norbert, *The Civilizing Process*, vol. I: *The History of Manners*, trans.
     Edmund Jephcott (Oxford, 1978)
——, *The Civilizing Process*, vol. II: *State Formation and Civilization*, trans. Edmund
     Jephcott with some notes and revisions by the author (Oxford, 1982)
Encyclopedia Judaica 1971, vol. VI (Jerusalem, 1971)
Englund, Peter, *Förflutenhetens landskap* (Stockholm, 1991)
Enzensberger, Christian, *Größerer Versuch über den Schmutz* (Munich, 1970)
Erasmus, Desiderius, *De civilitate morum puerilium* (Lugduni, 1536)
——, *The Ciuilitie of Childehode*, trans. Thomas Paynell (London, 1560)
Faryno, Jerzy, 'Neskol'ko obščih soobraženij po povodu konceptov "grjaznyj/
     čistyj"', *Studia Litteraria Polono-Slavica*, IV (1999), pp. 59–62
Fayet, Roger, 'Moderne Reinigung, postmoderne Kompostierung. Über ein
     abfalltheoretisches Modell und die eigentlichen Signaturen zweier Zeitalter',
     in *Verlangen nach Reinheit oder Lust auf Schmutz? Gestaltungskonzepte
     zwischen rein und unrein*, ed. Roger Fayet (Vienna, 2003), pp. 15–40
Franklin, Alfred, *La civilité*, vol. II (Paris, 1908)
Freud, Sigmund, 'Der Mann Moses und die monotheistische Religion', in
     Sigmund Freud, *Gesammelte Werke*, Band XVI: *Werke aus den Jahren
     1932–1939* (London, 1950), pp. 101–246
——, *Totem and Taboo*, authorized trans. by A. A. Brill (New York, 1946)
——, *Totem und Tabu*, in Sigmund Freud, *Gesammelte Werke*, Band IX
     (London, 1948)
——, *Das Unbehagen an der Kultur* (Vienna, 1930)
Friedell, Egon, *Kulturgeschichte des Altertums. Leben und Legende der
     vorchristlichen Seele*, Band I (Zurich, 1936)
Frykman, Jonas, 'Hel och ren. Kropp och tanke hos bönder och borgare',
     in *Den kultiverade människan*, ed. J. Frykman and O. Löfgren (Lund, 1979),
     pp. 131–220
Furuhjelm, Annie, *Den stigande oron* (Helsingfors, 1935)
Grammaticus, Saxo, *Danica historia libris XVI*, ed. Philippus Lonicerus (Frankfurt
     a.M., 1576)

Grönfors, Martti, 'Institutional Non-marriage in the Finnish Roma Community and Its Relationship to Rom Traditional Law', in *Gypsy Law: Romani Legal Traditions and Culture*, ed. Walter O. Weyrauch (Berkeley, CA, 2001), pp. 149–69

Hacker, P.M.S., *Appearance and Reality: An Investigation into Perception and Perceptual Qualities* (Oxford, 1991)

Hadot, Pierre, *Plotinus or the Simplicity of Vision* (Chicago, IL, 1998)

Hakamies, P., 'Karelische Sauna', *Rehabilitácia*, XVI (1982), Supplement 26–7, pp. 17–20

Hämäläinen, Nora, 'What is a Wittgensteinian Neo-Platonist?: Iris Murdoch, Metaphysics and Metaphor', *Philosophical Papers*, XLIII/2 (2014), pp. 191–225

Hänninen, Helena, *Puhtauden yhteiskunnallis-sosiaalisia ulottuvuuksia. Henkilökohtainen siisteys ja puhtaudenpito Keski-Suomessa noin 1890–1930*, MA dissertation (University of Jyväskylä, 1985)

Harpet, Cyrille, *Du déchet: Philosophie des immondices. Corps, ville, industrie* (Paris and Montreal, 1998)

Heidegger, Martin, *Being and Time*, trans. John Macquarrie and Edward Robinson (Oxford, 2001)

—, *Being and Time: A Translation of 'Sein und Zeit'*, trans. Joan Stambaugh (Albany, NY, 1996)

—, 'Das Ding', in Martin Heidegger, *Gesamtausgabe*, Band VII: *Vorträge und Aufsätze* (Frankfurt a.M., 2000), pp. 167–87

—, 'The Thing', in Martin Heidegger, *Poetry, Language, Thought*, trans. A. Hofstadter (New York, 1971), pp. 163–84

Heil, John, 'Real Tables', *Monist*, LXXXVIII/4 (2005), pp. 493–509

Heraclitus, 'Fragments of Heraclitus', trans. John Burnet (1912), available at https://en.wikisource.org/wiki/, accessed 16 October 2015

—, *Heraklit, Fragmente*, Greek and German, ed. Bruno Snell (Munich, 1926) Hesiod, 'Works and Days', in *Hesiod and Theognis*, trans. and intro. D. Wender (Harmondsworth, 1986), pp. 59–86

Hudgins, Andrew, 'Piss Christ – Andres Serrano 1987', *Slate*, 19 April 2000, www.slate.com/articles/arts/poem/2000/04, accessed 8 June 2016

Huizinga, Johan, *Homo ludens. Versuch einer Bestimmung des Spielelements der Kultur* (Amsterdam, 1994)

Huxley, Aldous, *Brave New World* [1932], www.idph.com, accessed 13 October 2015

Ingold, Tim, *Making: Anthropology, Archaeology, Art and Architecture* (London, 2013)

Järnefelt, Arvid, *Mitt uppvaknande* (Helsingfors, 1894)

Jokinen, Jami, 'Liasta näkyy vain osa', *Turkulainen*, 4 June 2003

Joutsivuo, Timo, 'Raamatun pitkäikäisyyden salaisuus', *Tieteessä tapahtuu*,
7 (2003), pp. 32–4

Kalman, Hildur, and Katarina Andersson, 'Framing of Intimate Care in Home
Care Services', *European Journal of Social Work*, XVII/3 (2014), pp. 402–14

Kant, Immanuel, *Critique of Pure Reason*, trans. Norman Kemp Smith
(London, 1964)

—, 'Mutmasslicher Anfang der Menschengeschichte', in Immanuel Kant, *Werke*,
Band IV: *Schriften von 1783–1788*, ed. Ernst Cassirer (Berlin, 1922), pp. 325–42

Keskiajan Turku – Det medeltida Åbo – Medieval Turku, Tourist brochure (Turku,
2001)

Kristeva, Julia, *Nations without Nationalism* (New York, 1993)

—, *Powers of Horror: An Essay on Abjection* (New York, 1982)

—, *Strangers to Ourselves* (New York, 1991)

Kross, Jaan, *The Czar's Madman: A Novel*, trans. Anselm Hollo (New York, 1993)

Krünitz, Johann Georg, *Ökonomisch-technologische Encyklopädie*, Band I (1773),
electronic publication of Universitätsbibliothek Trier, www.kruenitz.uni-trier.
de/1773, accessed 8 June 2016

Kuokkanen, Katja, 'Meuhkasiko markkinaväki keskiajalla?' *Turkulainen*,
24 July 2002

Lagerspetz, Olli, *Der Begriff Schmutz. Zum Verstehen unseres Zuhauses, unserer
Welt. Vom Autor autorisiert aus dem Schwedischen übertragen und redigiert
von Jürgen Birkle und Gerhard Schildberg-Schroth* (Berlin, 2015)

—, *Lika. Kirja maailmasta, kodistamme*, trans. Markus Lång (Helsinki, 2008)

—, *Smuts. En bok om världen, vårt hem* (Stockholm, 2006)

Langen, Ulrik, *Den afmægtige – en biografi om Christian 7* (Copenhagen, 2008)

Lapcic, M., 'Die Federn Richtung Himmel steigen lassen', *Frankfurter Allgemeine
Zeitung*, 27 October 2014

Laporte, Dominique, *History of Shit*, trans. Nadia Benabid and Rodolphe
el-Khoury, with an introduction by Rodolphe el-Khoury (Cambridge,
MA, 2000)

Le Corbusier [Charles-Edouard Jeanneret], *L'Art décoratif d'aujourd'hui, 1925*
(Paris, 2008)

Leddy, Thomas, 'Everyday Surface Aesthetic Qualities: "Neat", "Messy", "Clean",
"Dirty"', *Journal of Aesthetics and Art Criticism*, LIII (1995), pp. 259–68

—, *The Extraordinary in the Ordinary: The Aesthetics of Everyday Life*
(Peterborough, ON, 2012)

Leimu, P., 'Sauna as a Socializing Instrument', *Rehabilitácia*, XVI, Supplement 26–7
(1982), pp. 12–14

Levi, Primo, 'If This Is a Man', in Primo Levi, *If This Is a Man* and *The Truce*,
    trans. Stuart Woolf (London, 2007), pp. 15–179

Linn, Gudrun, 'Ur "Badrum och städning"', *Res Publica*, LVII (2002), pp. 21–9

Locke, John, *An Essay Concerning Human Understanding* (London, 1867)

'Loi ° 75–633 du 15 juillet 1975 relative à l'élimination des déchets et à la
    récupération des matériaux', *Journal officiel de la République française*
    (16 July 1975), p. 7279. Available at www.legifrance.gouv.fr, accessed
    5 July 2017.

Lowe, E. J., 'How are Ordinary Objects Possible?', *The Monist*, LXXXVIII/4 (2005),
    pp. 510–33

Lukes, Steven, *Émile Durkheim: His Life and Works* (Harmondsworth, 1973)

Lundgren, Gunilla, and Aljosha Taikon, *Aljosha - zigenarhövdingens pojke*
    (Stockholm 1998)

Luther, Martin, *The Table Talk of Martin Luther*, trans. and ed. William Hazlitt
    (London, 1872)

Lyttkens, Lorenz, *Den disciplinerade människan* (Stockholm, 1989)

McGinn, Colin, *The Meaning of Disgust* (Oxford, 2011)

Malmqvist, Ningtsu, *Ningtsus kinesiska kokbok* (Stockholm, 1988)

Mansikka, Tomas, 'Alkemisk uppbyggelselitteratur', *Finsk Tidskrift*, CCLI–CCLII
    (2002), pp. 397–408

Marx, Karl, *Capital*, vol. I, trans. Samuel Moore and Edward Aveling
    (New York, 1967)

——, 'Thesen über Feuerbach', in Karl Marx and Friedrich Engels, *Werke* (=MEW),
    Band III (Berlin, 1978), pp. 5–7

——, 'Theses on Feuerbach', trans. Cyril Smith, 1978, at www.marxists.org,
    accessed 8 June 2016

——, and Friedrich Engels, 'Die deutsche Ideologie', in Karl Marx and Friedrich
    Engels, *Werke* (=MEW), Band III (Berlin, 1978), pp. 9–521

Meløe, Jakob, 'Steder', *Hammarn*, 3 (1995), pp. 6–13

——, 'The Two Landscapes of Northern Norway', *Inquiry*, XXXI (1988), pp. 387–401

Midtgaard, Anna Magdalena L., 'The Dust of History and the Politics of
    Preservation', paper for the Nordic Summer University Winter Symposium,
    Circle 4: Information, Technology, Aesthetics, 3–5 March 2006, Helsinki

Miller, William Ian, *The Anatomy of Disgust* (Cambridge, MA, 1997)

Monem, Nadine, ed., *Dirt: The Filthy Reality of Everyday Life* (London, 2011)

Moos, Stanislaus von, 'Das Prinzip Toilette. Über Loos, Le Corbusier und
    die Reinlichkeit', *Verlangen nach Reinheit oder Lust auf Schmutz?*
    Gestaltungskonzepte zwischen rein und unrein, ed. Roger Fayet (Vienna,
    2003), pp. 41–58

Nandan, Y., *The Durkheimian School: A Systematic and Comprehensive Bibliography* (Westport, CT, 1977)

Nietzsche, Friedrich, *Der Wille zur Macht*, in Friedrich Nietzsche, *Werke*, Band XVI (Leipzig, 1911)

Nordström, Ludvig, 'Ur "Lort-Sverige"', *Res Publica*, LVII (2002), pp. 37–41

Nussbaum, Martha C., *Philosophical Interventions: Reviews, 1986–2011* (New York, 2012)

——, '"Secret Sewers of Vice": Disgust, Bodies, and the Law', in *The Passions of Law*, ed. Susan Bandes (New York, 1999), pp. 19–62

Nygård, Henry, *Bara ett ringa obehag? Avfall och renhållning i de finländska städernas profylaktiska strategier 1830–1930* (Åbo, 2004)

Osborne, Catherine, 'Heraclitus', in *Routledge History of Philosophy*, vol. I: *From the Beginning to Plato*, ed. C.C.W. Taylor (London, 1997), pp. 88–127

Pennanen, Kaisa, 'Humanistisesta paikan tulkinnasta ja lian käsitteestä', *Alue ja ympäristö*, III/1 (2004), pp. 55–61

Pico della Mirandola, Giovanni, *Oration on the Dignity of Man* (Chicago, IL, 1956)

Pitkänen, Leena, 'Sottakeittiö pelasti', *Turkulainen*, 23 August 2003, p. 12

Plato, *Parmenides*, in *The Dialogues of Plato*, trans. Benjamin Jowett (Chicago, IL, 1952), pp. 486–511

——, *The Republic*, in *The Dialogues of Plato*, trans. Benjamin Jowett (Chicago, IL, 1952), pp. 295–441

——, *The Sophist*, in *The Dialogues of Plato*, trans. Benjamin Jowett (Chicago, IL, 1952), pp. 551–79

Puranen, Clara, 'En anslående fest', in *Sagalund – 'min kostsamma leksak'*, ed. Li Näse, Sagalunds Museum (Kimito, 2000), pp. 8–43

Rousseau, Jean-Jacques, 'On the Social Contract', in Jean-Jacques Rousseau, *Basic Political Writings*, trans. Donald A. Cress (Indianapolis, IN, 1988), pp. 141–227

Rozin, Paul, and April E. Fallon, 'A Perspective on Disgust', *Psychological Review*, XCIV (1987), pp. 23–41

Rückert, Gertrud, 'Gedanken einer alten Frau zur allerletzten Seite der ZEIT', *Die Zeit*, 6 December 1994

Sahlberg, Irja, 'Byggnadsskick och heminredning', in *Kimitobygdens historia*, vol. II (Ekenäs, 1982), pp. 61–139

Sartre, Jean-Paul, *Being and Nothingness: An Essay on Phenomenological Ontology* (London, 1969)

——, *Nausea*, trans. Lloyd Alexander (New York, 1964)

——, *Sketch for a Theory of Emotions*, trans. Philip Mairet (London and New York, 1962)

——, 'Une idée fondamentale de la phénoménologie de Husserl: l'intentionnalité', in Jean-Paul Sartre, *La transcendance de l'ego, esquisse d'une description phénoménologique* (Paris, 1981), Appendix v, pp. 109–13

Scanlan, John, *On Garbage* (London, 2005)

Schmitt, Carl, *Der Begriff des Politischen. Text 1932 mit Vorwort und drei Corollarien* (Berlin, 1991)

Schwerhoff, Gerd, 'Zivilisationsprozess und Geschichtswissenschaft: Norbert Elias' Forschungsparadigma in historischer Sicht', *Historische Zeitschrift*, CCLXVI (1998), pp. 561–605

Searle, John, *Minds, Brains and Science* (Cambridge, MA, 1984)

Smith, William Robertson, *Lectures on the Religion of the Semites. First Series: The Fundamental Institutions* (London, 1974)

Solzhenitsyn, Alexander, *One Day in the Life of Ivan Denisovich*, trans. Ralph Parker (New York, 1963), www.kkoworld.com, accessed 31 May 2016

Spengler, Oswald, *Der Mensch und die Technik* (Munich, 1931)

——, *Der Untergang des Abendlandes*, Band I (Munich, 1921)

Sperring, Susanne, 'Han dokumenterade sitt smutsiga kök', *Åbo Underrättelser*, 14 August 2003

Strasser, Susan, *Waste and Want: A Social History of Trash* (New York, 1999)

Strohminger, Nina, 'The Meaning of Disgust: A Refutation', *Emotion Review*, VI/3 (2014), pp. 214–16

Suni, Timo, 'Tšuhnalainen automenodi', in *Toisten Suomi*, ed. Hannes Sihvo (Jyväskylä, 2001), pp. 196–242

Svenska Akademins ordbok (SAOB), http://g3.spraakdata.gu.se/osa/index.html, accessed 8 June 2016

Svensson, Per, *Svenska hem. En bok om hur vi bor och varför* (Stockholm, 2002)

Temsch, Jochen, 'Das wird schon wieder werden', *Die Zeit*, 25 November 1994

Theweleit, Klaus, *Male Fantasies*, vol. I, trans. Stephen Conway (Cambridge, 1987)

Thompson, Ewa Majewska, *Understanding Russia: The Holy Fool in Russian Culture* (Lanham, MD, 1987)

Tilander, Gunnar, *Stång i vägg och hemlighus. Kulturhistoriska glimtar från mänsklighetens bakgårdar* (Stockholm, 1968)

Törne, Elsa [Elna Tenow], *Renhet. En häfstång för den enskilde och samhället* (Stockholm, 1906)

Torrkulla, Göran, *Om mötet med konst som en dialektik mellan tilltal, gensvar och ansvar, eller om konsten som en dialogskapande vägkost*, lecture manuscript, Åbo Akademi University (Åbo, 2004)

Tyler, Imogen, 'Against Abjection', *Feminist Theory*, x (2009), pp. 77–98

——, *Revolting Subjects: Social Abjection and Resistance in Neoliberal Britain* (London, 2013)

Vilkuna, Kustaa, *Varsinais-Suomen kansanrakennukset. Varsinais-Suomen historia*, vol. II/1 (Porvoo, 1938)

Vuorela, Vilppu, *Kitchen Dreams*, exh. cat., Galleria Spectro, Turku (Turku, 2003)

Walker, A.D.M., 'The Ideal of Sincerity', *Mind*, LXXXVII, New Series (1978), pp. 481–97

Weil, Simone, *Lectures on Philosophy*, trans. Hugh Price, with an introduction by Peter Winch (Cambridge, 1993)

Wikipedia, 'James Croak', https://en.wikipedia.org, accessed 13 June 2016

Winberg, Christer, 'Några anteckningar om historisk antropologi', *Historisk tidskrift*, CVIII (1988), pp. 1–29

Winch, Peter, 'Understanding a Primitive Society', in Peter Winch, *Ethics and Action* (London, 1972), pp. 8–49

——, *The Idea of a Social Science and Its Relation to Philosophy* (London, 1958)

——, *Simone Weil: 'The Just Balance'* (Cambridge, 1989)

——, *Trying to Make Sense* (Oxford, 1987)

Wittgenstein, Ludwig, *Blue and Brown Books* (New York, 1965)

——, *Culture and Value*, ed. G. H. von Wright and Heikki Nyman, trans. Peter Winch (Chicago, IL, 1984)

——, *Notebooks, 1914–1916*, ed. G. H. von Wright and G.E.M. Anscombe, trans. G.E.M. Anscombe (New York, 1961)

——, *On Certainty* (New York, 1972)

——, *Philosophical Investigations*, ed. G.E.M. Anscombe and G. H. von Wright (Oxford 1953)

——, 'Remarks on Frazer's *Golden Bough*', in Ludwig Wittgenstein, *Philosophical Occasions, 1912–1951*, ed. James Klagge and Alfred Nordmann (Indianapolis, IN, 1993), pp. 115–55

Wolf-Knuts, Ulrika, 'Liktvättning', *Skärgård*, VII (1984), pp. 35–9

Wolkowitz, Carol, 'Linguistic Leakiness or Really Dirty? Dirt in Social Theory', in *Dirt: New Geographies of Cleanliness and Contamination*, ed. Ben Campkin and Rosie Cox (London, 2007)

ACKNOWLEDGEMENTS

Two other books by this author already exist with closely related contents and titles: the Swedish *Smuts. En bok om världen, vårt hem* (Stockholm, 2006; translation to Finnish 2008) and the German *Der Begriff Schmutz. Zum Verstehen unseres Zuhauses, unserer Welt* (Berlin, 2015). The two books are, however, not identical and the present work is not a direct translation of either. There are major additions, deletions and structural changes, complete chapters left out and added. Every single sentence has been reformulated and re-thought.

My Swedish book was a local success judging by the number and tone of newspaper reviews and invitations to talk shows in Sweden and Finland. It was certainly meant to be original research, not popular science. Still, I was much too aware of the implicit rules of academia to expect that a book on a theme of this kind – published in a vernacular to boot – would count towards anything in the university job market. But it is more to the point to mention those who have followed my work with interest and sympathy.

First of all my thanks go to Lars Hertzberg, my teacher, colleague and friend. His influence on my philosophical thinking has been continuous and often of a general character, which is why I hope Lars will excuse me for not giving the exact dates when I refer to remarks by him from discussions. I also thank my former teacher and colleague Hans Rosing, in particular for advice regarding the history of the scientific concept of matter. The participants at the philosophy research seminar at Åbo are acknowledged for their contributions to lively debates.

My colleague Gerhard Schildberg-Schroth raised the idea of producing a German version, translating and editing that work in close cooperation with Jürgen Birkle. In our final editing sessions we did not merely go through the translation, but we revised the very substance both in content, structure and style. In the present book, I have kept many of the solutions then arrived at. In this way, Gerhard has contributed greatly even to the shaping of the present English version.

The interdisciplinary character of this work has allowed me both to use my existing contacts within neighbouring disciplines and to make new ones.

Among these I wish at least to mention a few colleagues at Åbo Akademi University: Barbara Lönnqvist, Tomas Mansikka, Henry Nygård, Solveig Sjöberg-Pietarinen, Kirsti Suolinna, Göran Torrkulla, Bengt Kristensson Uggla and Anna-Maria Åström. Further, I extend my thanks to Karin Björkqvist, David Cockburn (of the University of Wales, Lampeter), Carita Lagerspetz, Mikko Lagerspetz, Jakob Meløe (of the University of Tromsø), Aleksander Motturi, Sören Stenlund (of the University of Uppsala), Lars Fredrik Svendsen (of the University of Bergen), as well as to Michael Leaman and other editors at Reaktion Books and to the anonymous reviewer for the present series.

The responsibility for any oddities or mistakes remains with the author. I do not suggest that any of the colleagues mentioned here would necessarily agree with what I have to say about the philosophy of dirt. That is the normal state of things in philosophy; not because philosophy is a fluffy subject but because philosophical inquiry always implies taking up a perspective on things – which is, by definition, *someone's* perspective.

No research funding was applied for or granted for the present volume. The earlier Swedish and German books received support from several sources, including the Åbo Akademi University Foundation.

This book is dedicated to the memory of my parents, with love and gratitude.